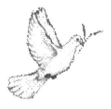

Hope

Hope when there is none
Hope when you're hurting
When you're angry
When you don't understand

There's a light at the end of the tunnel
And when you feel lost in the maze
And you don't know which way is forward or backwards
Don't give up

Help is on the way
Just like there's something bigger that kept you from knowing
There's something bigger that can come to your aid
Not just me, but the truth
The truth about Hope
There is

Christina Nevada

© <u>Healing Eczema</u> 1996-2009
by Christina Nevada

<u>Disclaimer</u>

This book was written for educational purposes only. Its contents are not intended to diagnose, treat or provide a second opinion on a health problem or disease. The information provided here is not medical advice and should not be taken as medical advice. Information must be recognized as personal opinion only. If you have questions concerning any topics in this document, you should seek the advice of a qualified professional.

TABLE OF CONTENTS

Thanks and Acknowledgements

Mishy, Sarah and Ryan,

Thank you for being the insurance policy on my life and giving me the will to live until I found hope.

Mom and Dad,

Thank you for praying for, caring for and guiding me.

Tony,

Thank you for giving me the tools to make this public.

Paul, Martha & Therese,

Thank you for your support.

God,

Thank you for pulling me out and teaching me and for giving me the desire to help other people with this. Every drop of blood I had with eczema is nothing compared to the blood you shed on the cross for me, and I love you.

.

All those who suffer from eczema,

You are my inspiration ... everything I do is for you.

ABOUT THE AUTHOR AND ECZEMA.NET

For 40 years I suffered with eczema. Decades of heavy topical cortisone use and dangerous levels of internal steroids didn't help me, and neither did the 20 antihistamines I was taking daily for the insane itch. It was torment, and I had lost all hope. By the grace of God and for the love of my three children, I didn't check off the planet. In despair, I became a self-employed, full time naturopathic eczema researcher and have been for nearly two decades.

As owner of www.eczema.net, just about all products for eczema were given to me for free, but none of them worked very well. You see, although two-thirds of people with eczema may benefit from merely topical therapies, one-third of eczema sufferers (as in my case) could see only a 15% improvement with topical treatments. I had to figure out what was going on inside.

It's about what you put on the skin, what you eat and the way you think (because stress also changes your biochemistry): it is ecology, not a defective body. You need to handle the skin on its terms and provide your body with the proper tools. I got well, and I can't credit one doctor, not one drug and not one product for my recovery. New research says most people that have eczema get it because they have thin skin. Let's examine this for a quick moment: they say you have eczema because your skin is thin, and for the last 57 years (since 1951) they have been giving you something to treat it (hydrocortisone) that thins the skin. That's not funny. I didn't want to become a dermatologist, because the western medicine philosophy couldn't help me. I also didn't want to become a naturopathic doctor, because I wanted only to specialize in eczema. We need to add to the training that dermatologists have, because it wasn't enough for me or for many others; but, I found out how to get well and so will you.

So how am I now in 2009? I'm excellent. My skin isn't sensitive anymore, and I can pretty much do whatever I want without too much care. A lot of my initial problem with eczema came after taking medicines like cough syrup that gave me rashes, and then I got more rashes from reactions to the medicines they gave me for the rashes. Right off the bat, I'd suggest you check out the list of drugs that cause rashes that's available on my web site, or call any pharmacy and ask if a rash can be a side effect from any medicine you're taking.

Since there are so many things you can do to improve eczema, the nice thing about it is that you don't need to be perfect but just want to head in the right general direction. After reading through my book, you won't be lost in a dark maze like a little blind mouse for decades like I was, but don't neglect getting tested to get answers.

My before and after photos of eczema can be viewed on my web site as well as other photos of eczema.

I. INTRODUCTION

This book was built from two decades of my naturopathic eczema research and the feedback of thousands of eczema sufferers from all over the world who contacted me through my web site: www.eczema.net.

This book is freely provided online, because I feel the need to do so for humanity. After so much suffering of my own while begging medical doctors for help that never came and still seeing the suffering of others, I am committed to freely providing this information.

Since this knowledge bank was built over the web, it was first written for web navigation and therefore organized in such a way that connected internal chapters together while containing links to many other web sites, supporting facts and documents. I've left much of the flavor of the web format here in this printed version so you can take this book, go to the same chapter online and then follow the supporting links there. To include here everything that's in the web site, I'd have to make this book well over 10,000 pages. With this format, although you'll find some repetitive facts, rather than to see it as a negative, I believe reinforcement is of great value in training. I am completely confident that you will have all the information you'll need in this printed book to recover from eczema, but know that there is a wealth of information in www.eczema.net attached to the online version of this book should you wish to refer to it.

The following is an article I wrote giving a brief overview of why eczema is occurring in perhaps a billion people worldwide.

Eczema and Body Ecology

All you want is the simple pleasure of having skin you can enjoy that feels soft and moves with you like silky clothing. To swim in the ocean, to play outside, to touch and hold your loved ones, to feel relaxed in it like others do ... the way it should be. Unfortunately, it isn't this way for millions of people. If drugs didn't cure you, doctors couldn't help you and hundreds of products out there failed, too, don't give up. You're not alone.

The National Institute of Health says over 15,000,000 Americans suffer from eczema, and US News and World Report says 10-20% of Americans suffer; however, considering The Census Bureau Pop Clock reporting January 2009 the US population at: 305,523,541 and the National Institute of Allergy and Infectious Disease's 30% figure, math suggests the actual figure in the USA alone is anywhere from 30 to 90 million. Australia also reports 30% of their population is suffering from eczema, and with the world's population at: 6,750,677,828 and a mid-zone 15% calculation, nearly 1 billion people worldwide may be suffering from some form or another of eczema. So uncomfortable, so much agony ... year after year. It's hard to get dressed much less go out, or swim or even touch people because it hurts. You've tried everything and nothing works ... and it's so unfair. I know, I've been there, and you can see my own before and after photos on www.eczema.net.

I became a pioneer in the field of naturopathic eczema research and have been a full-time, self-employed, naturopathic eczema researcher for nearly two decades. Not much of a living, mind you, because drug companies, western medicine doctors and eczema associations pretty much don't care about naturopathic medicine or helping me at all for that matter, because I disagreed with them. However, the good Dr. Alan Dattner, who heads up the American Academy of Dermatology's Task Force on Nutrition and Alternative Medicine wanted to co-publish this book with me; but, since my book was already written and since I want to give it away for free on the Internet, I released my book as a solo author. Nevertheless, I am honored by and publicly thank Dr. Dattner and do encourage you to go to holisticdermatology.com to see his work in this field as well. Further, the National Institute of Health asked me to help edit their very 1st Handbook on Atopic Dermatitis, so I did; but, since they are predominantly western medicine minded and I'm naturopathic, their book doesn't reflect my philosophy.

This book needed to be written to help share with people the other side of the untold eczema story--which does have a happy ending--a cure for eczema. It's called body ecology. Thousands of emails from eczema sufferers helped me write this book as I studied biochemistry, diet and ecology centering all my research around eczema ... and just about every single product for eczema was given to me for free to try.

I haven't found this much information specializing in eczema any other place in the world, and you should be confident that there are many people who have recovered from eczema with the information provided in this book. So let's begin ...

What Eczema Is

Eczema is a general term used to describe a variety of rashes where the skin may be itchy, red & inflamed, weepy or blistering, dry, scaly and thickened. Although eczema can develop any place on the body, it typically appears on the hands, wrists, arms, neck, upper chest, face and backs of knees. It is not contagious.

It is characterized as an immune system disorder (atopy). However, recent scientific research indicates that two-thirds of people with eczema may be suffering from merely contact dermatitis (a form of eczema) adding that most people get eczema from having thin skin. Think about this: they now say you have eczema because you have thin skin, yet for last 57 years, since 1951, they have been giving you something to treat it that thins the skin: cortisone. That's not funny, but thank goodness sunlight, Gotu Kola and other hormones, among other things, help re-thicken the skin.

For the other one-third of eczema sufferers, there's something else going on inside the body, so there can only be a 15% improvement with topical products and the remainder 85% improvement has to come from internal changes. Reality is that most doctors and dermatologists don't know how to teach you how to change your body's biochemistry, because they get less than 1 semester of nutrition in medical school. It's like psychiatrists who are trained to give drugs, but psychologists who are trained to teach you how to change your thinking so you can get well. You thought since you didn't get well that they were right: no cure, after all, it's on drug television commercials. Think again ...

Why Eczema

Externally Speaking

The #1 drug prescribed is hydrocortisone ointment, but even eczema can be aggravated by the use of hydrocortisone, petrolatum, neomycin & diphenhydramine. Most problems come from the use of harsh or sensitizing chemicals on the skin, including soap. The skin's barrier function can get damaged from the use of soap, because skin is supposed to be slightly acidic, and most soaps are alkaline. It's the skin's natural acid mantle and good bacteria living on the skin that protect us from harmful bacteria; so, remember, don't try and kill all your bacteria. There's nothing better than the real thing in terms of your own natural oils anyway. Besides, water is a cleanser, and you can wash most areas with just water most of the time. If you use more, though, aim for something pH balanced like Dove, Aquaderm or Cetaphil. Generally speaking, though, cleansers need only be used under the arm pits, soles of the feet and the groin area. There's a great article on the pH of different soaps and their effects on the skin in my site. I like to use lemon, milk, yogurt, honey or even oil sometimes.

Laundry soap residue left in clothes can also irritate the skin. So, just use one-third of the amount recommend, and you might not have to double rinse your clothing anymore. I learned that from an appliance repairman who says dishwasher and laundry detergent manufacturers recommend using way too much soap, and that's not good for the machines and leaves soap residue behind on your dishes, your clothing ... and your skin.

Regarding soap and staph, and acne for that matter, soap residue is one of unfavorable bacteria's favorite foods. While we're on the subject of acne, drying agents for acne can actually stimulate the sebaceous glands to make more oil, because they tell your oil glands that your face is dry and so it tries to make more oil. In the same way, did you ever wonder what putting oil on your skin for years is telling your oils glands? I wish to make products that stimulate your oil glands to produce more oil: androgens (male hormones) stimulate your oil glands to make more oil, and hydrocortisone hinders the production of oil ... imagine that. More importantly, I wish to emphasize that you should try to keep your natural oils.

See, also, the Calcium section for its important role in the barrier function..

Internally Speaking

Have you ever asked a dermatologist if hormones have anything to do with eczema, and the answer you got was, "no." Tell me then, why is the number one treatment for eczema corticosteroids (hormones)? Later, you'll join me on an adventure into the wide world of hormones as they pertain to eczema and the skin. You're in for a wonderfully amazing trip and discovery.

This next brief section gets a little technical, but don't worry if it seems like a foreign language to you right now, because most of this book is an easy read, and you don't need to get bogged down with understanding the underlying mechanisms as I will break it down later and make it very simple for you.

Many people with atopic eczema have adequate or elevated levels of linoleic acid (omega-6 or "LA") but deficiencies in Gamma linolenic acid ("GLA") and DGLA. There's a problem in the metabolism of essential fatty acids--a reduced rate of activity of the enzyme delta 6-desaturase that converts linoleic acid to GLA and alpha-linolenic acid to stearidonic acid. Such reduced activity is due to a mutation of, altered expression of, change in cofactors required for the presence of, or inhibitors of: enzymes.

Reduced conversion of LA to its metabolites and reduced rate of incorporation of essential fatty acids ("EFAs") into phospholipids leads to a reduced formation of prostaglandin E1 (PGE1) which in turn leads to lower concentrations of cyclic AMP and to a selective hyperactivity of parts of the immune system. Therapeutically, GLA increases the production of anti-inflammatory prostaglandins, which decreases itching. Studies report that patients treated with GLA exhibit less inflammation, dryness, scaling. In one study, low dose GLA therapy reduced the severity of skin lesions by 30%, whereas higher doses resulted in a 43% improvement.

The digestion and absorption of fats, including GLA, takes place in the small intestine in the gastrointestinal tract with the action of lipase enzymes and bile salts. Bile contains lecithin, which emulsifies fats into small droplets. This increases the surface area so that enzymes secreted from the pancreas can digest fats in the duodenum. EFA deficiency can be reversed with lipase. Individuals who ingest supplemental GLA are advised to take additional antioxidants, especially vitamin E, to protect against free radical oxidation in the body.

Note also that zinc is necessary for at least two stages in EFA metabolism, the conversion of linoleic acid to gamma-linolenic acid, and the mobilization of dihomogammalinolenic acid (DGLA) for the synthesis of 1 series PGs.

Fatty Acid Transport in the Lymphatic System

Lymph vessels are present in the lining of the gastrointestinal tract. While most other nutrients absorbed by the small intestine are passed onto the portal venous system to drain via the portal vein into the liver for processing, fats are passed onto the lymphatic system to be transported to the blood circulation via the thoracic duct. The nutrients that are released to the circulatory system are processed by the liver, having passed through the systemic circulation. The lymph system is a one-way system, transporting interstitial fluid back to blood. Basically, the lymphatic is the body's filter system which supports immune function.

A healthy lymphatic system filters out bacteria and other foreign particles. Lymphatics clear the spaces between our cells and carry away toxins and foreign particles such as bacteria, large proteins, cholesterol and viruses. We were taught that the liver and kidneys clear away toxins, but it is actually the lymphatics that clear away the fluid that bathes each cell of our body. The white cells, called lymphocytes, circulate in and out of the lymphatics and help destroy foreign particles like bacteria, viruses and parasites.

Some trouble begins when the lymphatic system becomes blocked or the flow of lymph slows down appreciably. It's like the kitchen sink: if the drain is clogged but you leave the water running, the water will eventually run all over the floor. Not only can the lymphatic fluid be blocked, but so can all the toxins, bacteria and viruses that the lymphatic fluid normally drains from the body. It is no surprise that lymphedema patients suffer from other health ailments. The stagnant lymph fluid is a breeding ground for bacteria, parasites and viruses and a cesspool of toxic waste. The lymphatics are an integral part of our immune system.

The good news is that regular exercise and jumping or using a mini-trampoline are one of the best treatments your lymphatic system can receive and are great and fun ways to detoxify the body. So ... JUMP!! Jump for health and jump for joy ... also because this technical section is over. (smiles)

You see, it's a wonderful nutritional orchestra, and get this: 75% of your beautiful immune system is found in your gastrointestinal tract where 3 ½ pounds of bacteria naturally and normally reside.

Bacteria and Enzymes

Among other things, good bacteria known as probiotics assist in digestion, enzyme production (including lipase enzymes) and B vitamin production that aid in the metabolism of fats. When the balance of bacteria is off, so is digestion, including the metabolism of fats. To understand this fully, you'll need to see the Bacteria section.

Remember we mentioned that lecithin emulsifies fats? Well, inositol and choline combine to produce lecithin, a type of lipid that is needed to form healthy membranes for every living cell in the body. So, how does the body produce inositol? You got it: bacteria. Bacteria in the intestines convert the phytic acid into inositol, so the body is able to manufacture its own supply. Note: Bacteria produce hundreds of different enzymes, including amylase whose deficiency has also been implicated in eczema.

Since some people with eczema may have trouble breaking down fats, consider starting out with powders or liquids as opposed to probiotics that are encapsulated in oil unless you are taking a lipase enzyme to break down the oil so that you can get the benefit of the probiotic that is encapsulated within the oil.

Immune System Memory and Glyconutrients

Since the immune system has memory, immune system modulators such as glyconutrients that address hypersensitivity and immune system memory may reverse immunologic abnormalities and their effects on the skin. Glyconutritionals modulate or "regulate" the immune system. This means that they correct an overactive immune system and boost an underactive immune system. See: "How Do Glyconutrients Work?"

Some natural sources of glyconutrients are: echinacea, aloe vera, honey, cocoa, coconut, licorice, sarsaparilla, garlic, onions, mushrooms, soybeans, whey protein, chestnuts, bovine and shark cartilage, broccoli, pumpkin, brussel sprouts, avocado, carrots, cauliflower, celery, cucumber, potato, asparagus, lettuce, spinach, peas, okra, corn, green beans, capsicum, cabbage, eggplant, tomatoes, turnip, guava, pears, blackberries, raspberries, grapes, bananas, mangoes, cherries, strawberries, apples, apricot, cherries, cranberries, dates, nectarine, peaches, pears, pineapple, plums, prunes … just to name some. You can search more for "natural sources of glyconutrients" on the Internet using Google.

Diet, Detoxification and Internal pH

Regarding our diet and infant formulas, internally the human body should be slightly alkaline with the ideal pH being 7.35. Did you know that metabolic acidosis is common in babies fed cows' milk-based formula and that eczema can be an emergency expulsion of acid toxins through the skin? If we are too acidic inside, we can get sick, and this may be one reason why 10% of all infants have eczema or suffer from colic. Infants need an alkaline formula, and we all need to be alkaline internally. For that matter, if mom is acidic, so may baby's breast milk be. You will read more about this in the Alkalizing section and more about infant formula in the Child and Infantile Eczema section.

Drinking enough unchlorinated water to hydrate from within, along with taking your good fats like fish, borage and flax oil, as well as glucosamine, will help the skin retain moisture. Moreover, when I started drinking milk again, I didn't suffer from dry skin in the winter anymore. Go figure that one out, because I can. The one thing physicians told me stay away from, milk, was what helped me a lot because of the calcium, and you'll read more about why in the Calcium section. To rebuild the skin, you need protein/amino acids and vitamins and minerals. Remember that good bacteria break down foods for absorption in the body.

Recall how we talked about the lymphatic system to detoxify and clean the body? Well, the skin is the largest eliminative organ. Cleaning the body on the inside is very helpful in reducing the allergic (atopic) component, and greens like kale and parsley can help do that and are well known for helping atopic dermatitis, too, so juice, blend, drink and eat them.

Food allergies and certain foods such as dairy, wheat, gluten (glue up your insides) and nuts can trigger eczema outbreaks in some people, but probiotics significantly help with food allergies, too, and thank goodness for that. Hydrochloric acid deficiencies as well as overproduction of candida (yeast) may also be associated; but, cheer up, because you guessed it, good bacteria address these as well, since probiotics help produce B vitamins that help produce hydrochloric acid, and probiotics also plug up the holes of leaky gut and fight candida ... and all that is why I'm a huge advocate of good bacteria. These are some of your best friends. Later we'll talk how bacteria can prevent eczema and asthma in your unborn children with research from NIH.

In Sum

Nutrition, detoxification, anti-stress coping skills and external practices are all a part of healing eczema. The body is trying to tell you something, and it isn't just a defective on/off switch in the inflammatory cycle and may not be just a damaged barrier function. Inflammation is the process that fights infection; and, if there is a bacterial or fungal over-colonization like staphylococcus aureus, steroids--which stop the inflammation process--will make the problem worse by allowing infection to run wild and further thin the skin damaging even more the barrier function. Changing your body's chemistry internally and externally to provide the proper environment for skin health will bring about a permanent change in this condition ... and that's the cure for eczema. It is ecology.

Finally, you'll notice that I don't address every kind of therapy like acupuncture or photo and urine therapy, but that doesn't mean I don't see value in other therapies. There's some good in everything, it's just that I don't want needles stuck in me, I didn't enjoy sunburn itch on top of eczema itch, and I don't want to drink urine to stimulate cell mediated immunity or put it all over myself like other cultures have found helpful. Everybody needs to do whatever it is they feel good about doing, and we don't all like apples now, do we, so thank goodness for oranges, too (smile) ... what I mean is that the nice thing about all this is that since there are so many things you can do to improve your condition, there is no one right way or need for perfection, and that, my dears, is science.

II: BE ENCOURAGED

A little boy was told by his teacher in school that he couldn't touch the toys there anymore, because his hands were too bloody from eczema. While the other children played, he was told to go watch TV instead. His mom emailed me out of desperation asking for help. I was so glad she did, because it was only a few weeks later when she emailed me back to tell me her little boy is recovering from his eczema. She wrote,

> *"His hands are getting a lot better. His palms used to be raw and scaly and are now normal palms, and his fingers seem to be getting better everyday."*

Here are just some of the physician recommendations and hundreds of testimonials I've received that I'd like you to see and be encouraged by. For the top 100 Testimonials, you can go to www.eczema.net.

Medical Book Reviews

"Stellar advice." Former Managing Editor of Prevention Magazine and author of Alternative Cures - **Bill Gottlieb**

"This book on eczema is packed with information to help patients with eczema find their way through the multitude of environmental and dietary exposures which are likely to aggravate the condition." **Dr. Alan Dattner.** *Dr. Dattner holds a 40-year background in Cellular Immunology and founded and heads up the American Academy of Dermatology's Task Force on Nutrition and Alternative Medicine.*

"A great and very informative web site." **Understand.com**

"Thanks to you I was able to become a human again. I have suffered from this since birth (37 years), but the last 5 years were unbelievable. My family and I cannot thank you enough. I am a registered nurse, a medical student and a doctor of natural medicine, and nothing had helped me as much as your protocol." **Roberto D'Lorm, RN, MSII, NMDsIII**

"What a great knowledge bank of hints, facts, and common sense ideas. Your book is a reflection of the ideas and lessons I have been trying to give to my patients for 20+ years. It's just nice to see it compiled in one place so well. Thank You". **C. Steven Smith MS/MD FAAAI, Board Certified, Allergist/ Immunology, 1017 DuPont Square North, Louisville, Kentucky 40207**

"I am happy to note that you are educating people with eczema". **Prof. Dr. M. Srinivasulu, M.Sc.(Psy.), M.D (K.C.), Ph.D (N.I.A.) Andhrapradesh, INDIA**

"Your site is awesome. Am referring a client to it. thanks so much for sharing your experience and all the info!" **Prem, MD**

"I am also a researcher and sufferer of eczema and have found your site brilliant and very helpful !! I will spread the word of your website!!" **Carolyn**

"An excellent source for information on eczema." **Boyce N. Berkel, M.D.**

"I cannot congratulate you highly enough for the invaluable information you provide in your web site. I am also a medical researcher ... I wish you continued success in your remarkable work." **Douglas**

18

"I truly enjoyed your website. I think you have a very good perspective of the disease process. I appreciate all the work that you have gone through. I can say this, until you suffer through this yourself, one does not have any concept of the suffering one has. I am a gastroenterologist. Thanks again for the website. I'm sure it has helped many." **Joe**

Testimonials

"I was once described by a team of dermatologists as the worst cast they had seen. I've learned more from you than I have from the dozen or so doctors and derms I've dealt with over the past 20 years. My condition has dramatically improved ... thanks to you." **Chad**

"How can I thank you enough???? I thank God the day that I read your book!!! After suffering from eczema for 56 years, I thought there was no hope anymore. After reading your book and making some changes, my eczema is gone!!!! I never in my wildest dreams thought that it could happen. I don't scratch at night at all, whereas before I would wake up, bleeding, and then would end up with a staph infection. My whole life has changed, I am not miserable anymore..... Friends and family cannot believe it is the same me. so, I thank you from the bottom of my heart for all of your hard work, putting this book together and I have spread the word to other eczema sufferers. Doctors can all get on a slow boat to China, as far as I am concerned !!! Thank you again, you are an angel . Your friend always," **Judy**

"This book sets the benchmark for information on this disease that's so hard to cope with sometimes. This is coming from a life time sufferer." **Corey**

"Your insights literally changed our family's life -- our 10 year old has/had atopic dermatitis for nine years until we found your web site." **Nancy**

"I was so happy to find your site! I've suffered my entire life, and this is the most comprehensive source of information I've come across." **Judith**

"Thank you so much for all the information. I've suffered all my life (20 years) and haven't heard of half the treatments that you teach." **Laura**

"I have had eczema for 39 years and have seen every specialist in Washington, DC and Baltimore, MD ... your book to date is the best.!!!" **Rose**

"Until finding you site I was living in agony. I have improved dramatically! Everything you have recommended to me has worked. I just wanted to tell you how much you have helped me. You have changed my life!" **Marissa**

"I wish I had access to your information much sooner. Your style of writing is very comprehensive. It has been very informative and helpful. Much more than all the doctors and specialists I've seen put together." **Grover**

"I have had this disease for 21 years. Your book is like fresh air for me. I'm getting better since I follow your advice. I wanted to thank and congratulate your efforts." **Patricia**

"My 7 year old son had a severe case for three years. We went to many dermatologists, allergists, doctors, clinics, etc., and they gave us no hope. None at all. After reading your book, he is almost totally clear. Thank you so much. You cannot believe (or maybe you can) the horrible time we have had the past 3 years." **Cathy**

"First, let me thank you. My three year old sister has dermatitis, and your book has been more informative than the doctors we have taken her to or the books we have consulted." **Michael**

"My daughter is 5 years old and has suffered with this horrible disorder since she was two. You have been a miracle for me." **Jennifer**

"I'm 17 and have suffered since infancy ... excruciating. What you're doing is amazing. I think you know more about this than anyone ever has. I'm better off for having found your book." **Rob**

"I have been able to find absolutely no relief until I read your book." **Curtis**

"Excellent. I have had dermatitis all my 36 years and have figured out a lot along the way, but I have found your book extremely informative." **Michael**

"I want to thank you for such an informative book. I have suffered for about 4 years. The countless doctors and dermatologist I have seen never told me anything but gave me medication that didn't work. I didn't realize that I was causing the flare ups until reading your book. And by using your suggestions, I rarely have a flare up; but, when I do I use your remedies and they work like a charm." **Shannon**

"There are lots of things I learned reading your book that the dermatologist never mentioned." **Veronica**

"Thank you so much. After suffering for 15 years I have finally been able to control it and understand it better." **Alvaro**

"You are a life saver - thanks for a fantastic book. The work you have put into creating this is amazing." **Rose**

"I just wanted to let you know that I cleared up within about 3 days of reading and following your advice. Mine was pretty severe and painful." **George**

"I use to itch unbearably. It affected my entire life and I always felt self conscious. Now, the itching has deteriorated thanks to the wonderful info you provide." **Jake**

"It amazes me how much there is to learn. I've suffered for about 10 years now, and have never seen or heard of such a comprehensive guide of tips and references. Surely the dermatologists are running scared!" **Kevin**

"Thank you again (like all those who have written in your testimonials) for all the information that you have provided. As a severe sufferer like yourself for over 30 years, I have tried some of the things that you mentioned but have learned a lot more here." **Kath**

"Congratulations for the accuracy of the information ... it is the best information about atopic dermatitis you can find. All allergy doctors should read it." **Jose**

"I found this book so informal and thorough. It's amazing what they won't or don't have the time to say at the doctors." **Brenda**

"This has been the most helpful resource I've seen on the subject." **Matt**

"Your book is the most definitive and helpful book." **Yasser Kassana, UK**

"I'm overwhelmed at the amount of solid information! Have you been on the talk show circuit yet? You'd be a great ambassador of those of us with this disease to the millions who don't know what it is or how to cure it." **Kevin**

"I must state that it is truly wonderful what Christina has done in authoring this excellent book. She has given hope to many people who have despaired (and given up all hope) after conventional dermatology had failed them." **John**

"This is fantastic. As a long time sufferer, it has given me a whole new slant on my problem. Makes the whole Internet worthwhile." **Julius**

"I just want to thank you so, so much for your wonderful site with tons of information and for your hard work getting this information! ... and I couldn't believe that you give all this information for free! I mean starting from February I got a very bad case of eczema that lasted for nearly two months and was getting worse every day. I have had eczema since my childhood, and now I'm 26. It seems it only gets worse with age and not better as many of the doctors were saying. Usually I don't have it in summer but would have bad outbreaks in autumn and spring and usually on my wrists, palms, face and neck. This year it was the worst case ever. I did not know what to do. I started looking on the Internet. Mostly as you know they all offer some "miracle" cream, but I did not believe all that as I felt somehow that this condition must come from within. I was astonished when I found your site ... so much information ... all of which made so much sense. I finally started to understand what I am dealing with. I kept reading and reading. I could not believe my eyes. I started following all your advice, got good probiotics (Udo's choice), fish oils, enzymes, calcium with magnesium, good multivitamins,

especially for skin and hair, gotu kola and apple cider vinegar. I started to salt my food with organic sea salt, and of course I started following the alkaline diet. You know what ... my horrible eczema, all the red patches and crusts disappeared in about 10 days. I could literally see improvement every day more and more. Wow! I'm just sorry I did not take before and after pictures of my wrists and arms! You would not believe this is the same person! Moreover, the skin on my face never felt like this before: it is like if the skin became thicker, before it was quite fragile. It's so smooth! I experimented for 5 days and did not wash my face or put any moisturizer on it. You would expect the skin would feel dry, gray, unhealthy looking, right? Well, my face never looked and felt so luminous, moisturized and pleasant to touch. Wow ... unbelievable! Christina, THANK YOU AGAIN! for literally giving me my life back! Keep up the good work and new researches on the subject! With great respect," **Natalia**

III. PROPER PERSPECTIVE

If you remember anything, remember this: We are biochemically different; and, since there are so many things we can do to improve our condition, it is not about the overwhelming number of things we have to do, it's about the seemingly limitless choices of wonderful things we can do. It isn't about being a perfectionist, it's about the gift of knowledge of ecology and our body's ability to heal itself. Little by little, just by taking little baby steps, you will learn to change your biochemistry and recover. It is going to be okay, and you can relax and experience great freedom on your journey of recovery.

Some of the following information has been previously touched upon in my "Eczema and Body Ecology" article you just read, but I've revisited some matters here in this section to allow for concept reinforcement before we break everything down in the remainder of the book.

Eczema is a general term used to describe a variety of skin rashes. These rashes are from any or a combination of these: not drinking enough water, an imbalance of bacteria, improper internal or external pH, digestive issues, drug and food sensitivities or allergies, a need to detoxify, nutrition, external chemical destruction, stress and hormonal imbalances. No worries, though, because addressing any one of these can improve your condition, so it's not about having to do everything, it's more like: Wow !! Look how many things I can do to get better !! (smiles) The body is an amazing and miraculous thing.

Generally, some chemicals we come in contact with can disturb or destroy the pH balance of our skin. For example, alkaline soaps remove the acid mantle, and the acid mantle is what protects the skin from bad bacteria and fungus. When the acid mantle is disturbed, the natural protection against harmful bacteria and fungal colonization is reduced, and with reduced protection, the skin can become more vulnerable to sensitization and infection. Too much staph can be common in people with eczema, so that's why it's important to get tested for staph.

We need to detoxify (clean out our insides), provide the right balance of bacteria, pH and nutrients.

Stress can also aggravate eczema, and I'll show you the mechanisms of why and what do to about it later. One thing I'd like to say now, though, is healthy boundaries in relationships is huge. There's a book and video series I love called Boundaries by Henry Cloud and John Townsend which can be found at: cloudtownsend.com. You'll also find free short videos on depression, anxiety, loneliness and many more psychological topics. I can't stress going there enough. ☺

It's an orchestra. We need to change the way we handle chemicals, food and people. It is going to be okay, because with my help, you will beat this. Scientists are actually working on nanobots to interact with our biological neurons to have immortality within the next 20 to 30 years … now that's amazing!!

As wonderfully engineered as our bodies are, ecology isn't something new. You can get well, and now you can understand why, so don't believe doctors who don't know about nutrition or drug company commercials when they say there is no cure ... or any institution that spends more money on drug research and development than on prevention. I didn't believe them when they told me there's no cure, and my recovery and this book is the result of not giving up, so don't you give up either. The information in this book has helped thousands of people who the doctors couldn't help, and I believe with all my heart that it will help you, too. Take it from a former severe eczema sufferer who wants to give this all away for free.

The Majority of Problems

Skin care products, hair preparations (including colors which are extremely alkaline), and facial makeup account for the majority of problems in people who suffer from contact dermatitis which is the #1 form of eczema.

New Research Article

"New Eczema Research Revolutionizes Understanding of the Condition" Los Angeles (PRWEB) October 24, 2006. **The National Skin Care Institute.**

Their article says most people get eczema because they have thin skin. I've quoted their article in italics and inserted my comments throughout.

Scientists have long believed that eczema is an allergic reaction. However, new research has found that most eczema cases are the result of an entirely different phenomenon – a defective skin barrier that predisposes eczema sufferers to damage from environmental irritants. These findings revolutionize scientists' understanding of eczema and open the door to more effective eczema treatment.

I am glad that scientists are saying that chemical irritants are the #1 cause of eczema (that's hopeful and good news). However, it is misleading to use the terms "defective skin barrier" and "predisposes," because it is like saying cars have a predisposition to crash, and when they get damaged in a crash, it is the car's defect.

Hundreds of dermatologists are now recommending the use of a shielding lotion, a new type of skin care product that mimics the skin's protective outer layer. This may well be the new global standard for eczema treatment.

Occlusive barriers are not good for long term use, because they suffocate the skin. Better to protect the skin from the chemical damage of soaps, lotions, shampoos and chlorinated water than to suffocate the skin and continue to expose the skin to damaging chemicals.

The new study, published in the Journal of Allergy and Clinical Immunology, revealed surprising findings - the raised allergic antibodies that would support the immune reaction theory were not present in two-thirds of the cases studied.

Although 2/3rds may be suffering from purely contact dermatitis, still, 1/3rd remain with raised allergic antibodies indicating that the immune system is involved. The public has already been told they have a defective off/on switch in the inflammatory cycle and that there is no cure. Now, they are told they have a defective barrier function. Damaged barrier function and immune response, yes ... defective, I don't think so. One implies they are genetically defective and a condition with which they must permanently live; the other implies something ecologically altered their body's response and that by addressing the root of the problem they can recover. I believe eczema is from ecological disturbances within the body and on the skin's surface and that once these disturbances are corrected, the sufferer will recover. I say blame it on the chemicals and imbalances and not on the human body.

Instead, they found evidence that the protective surface layer of the skin was compromised. Scientists now believe that this problem is the true source of many eczema conditions and that treatment must take an abrupt turn away from the immune system focus towards preserving the integrity of the skin's protective layer.

Of course the barrier function is compromised with alkaline soaps, fragrances, preservatives and chemical sensitizers that are found in the average household. Even chlorinated water may dry out the skin and harm the skin's barrier functions. How many people let household cleaning chemicals touch their skin when the label says don't.

The profound news of the impact of probiotics on the immune system with regard to eczema never even saturated the eczema community before studies like this get widely published saying scientists should bail out on the immune research ship. For me, that's a problem.

Scientists suspect that the breakdown is due to a combination of factors - a genetic predisposition to thin skin which is then easily damaged by moisture loss and irritation caused by overheating, cold weather, dry winds and exposure to chemical irritants like soap or detergents. One thing is certain, while thin skin is more susceptible to developing eczema, exposure to irritants is often the key precipitating element for flares.

According to Dr. Peter Helton, cosmetic dermatologist and medical director of the Helton Skin and Laser Institute in Newport Beach, California, "In order for the skin to heal and return to its healthy condition you have to seal in the moisture and oils that are below the outer layer of skin and protect it from the irritants in the environment."

Although some irritants are named, the way they think still puts the blame on the skin and not on the irritating chemicals; but, yes, in order for the skin to heal, it is crucial to protect it, and occlusive barriers like mineral oil are great temporary band-aids to help do that.

A good shielding lotion does just that. "Shielding lotions can significantly restore the skin's natural barrier and thus make it less susceptible to environmental irritants and eczema flares," explains Dr. Lisa Benest, a board certified dermatologist in Burbank, California. A recent Transepidermal Water Loss (TEWL) study found that shielding lotion increases the protective layer formation properties by more than 50 percent within one hour of application. "A shielding lotion is a new kind of lotion. It is a new technology that blends moisturizers with a light silicone material that is like a liquid film that bonds with the surface of your skin. It is like wearing an invisible shield that helps heal the skin. It keeps the moisture in and keeps the irritants out," said Dr. Helton.

It takes four days for barrier functions to return to normal after they have been damaged with chemical irritants and thirty days for all layers of the skin to rejuvenate; so, if consumers continue to wash away their natural acid mantle and good bacteria and dissolve their intercellular cement with hot soapy water, they'll be in the damaged barrier function boat forever. For the two-thirds with merely contact dermatitis, understand that urine is better for your skin than soap. You can use yogurt to wash your skin, so do protect your skin from chemicals and sensitizers.

Learn about the huge value of calcium in this regard. Read, also, about how red palm oil and sunflower oil can repair the barrier function and how topical olive and soybean oils delay repair.

For those who think it is more than contact dermatitis, continue to explore probiotics, but don't stress about it, because there's so much we can do using nutrition to get better.

> *Steroid creams and ointments are the traditional topical eczema treatment, but, as they can further damage the protective layer, these new findings indicate the need for a different approach. Shielding lotion may be the wave of the future.*

First the experts give you topical steroids that thin the skin, and then they tell you that you got the condition because you have thin skin … and we still look at them as the experts? (lol) The good news is that the sunlight, Gotu Kola and other hormones are just some of the things that will help re-thicken the outer layer of the epidermis.

I'm not saying don't ever use topical steroids because sometimes they, especially betamethasone valerate can be helpful;

however, if you live off of them, you can learn so much here so that you don't need to.   Just think about being easy on your skin, and I'll describe for you shortly a little more in detail your skin's barrier function as well as how hormones affect the thickness and oil production of the skin.

Different Folk Remedies for Different Folks

What irritates my skin might not irritate yours, and vice versa. Why?   Everyone is bio-chemically different.   Different environments, quantities and interactions of carbohydrates, fats, proteins, enzymes, vitamins, minerals, fiber and differences in the way our bodies perform, such as one end-organ response to another account for why we react differently when exposed to the same thing.   So, even though some things can irritate eczema, concerning one's self with them all is unwarranted. You must reinforce this protective truth in your mind: a few simple changes can make all the difference.

Most Importantly and Always Remember

Whatever you do, don't panic because it's downhill from here, and don't stop believing you can get better.   Remember I'm available for consultations, and we can use the free internet calling software Skype to talk internationally.   Go to www.skype.com to download it, and my username is: ChristinaNevada.

IV. EXTERNAL CONSIDERATIONS

Okay, so now that we have a bird's-eye view, let's break it all down and make it really simple for you.

Acid Mantle

The skin--by a secretion of sweat and oil glands--makes a protective film on the skin's surface that inhibits the growth of bacteria, fungi, and other microorganisms. It is a natural defense barrier and is called the acid mantle, and the normal pH should range from 4.5 to 6.5.pH (potential of hydrogen) refers to the degree of acidity or alkalinity.

The pH scale goes from 0 to 14

> ➢ Neutral is 7
> ➢ Lower than 7 is acidic
> ➢ Above 7 is alkaline (or basic)

Most soaps are alkaline (9.5-11), and these alkaline substances remove our acid mantle. Eczematous skin tends to have raised pH and cannot easily return to an acid pH after washing with soap, so cleaning substances that are almost neutral (pH 6-7) are best for the skin. Here's a very interesting article on the pH of different soaps and their effects on the skin that says the

Dove bar, Aquaderm and Cetaphil cleansers have a slightly acidic pH of 6 which is good to use on the skin.

Alkaline hair products are one reason people have scalp and ratty hair issues, but we'll talk more about that in the <u>Hair</u> section.

More information about pH and using water externally is found in the <u>External Water</u> section.

Soap Damage

Many people think their natural oils and bacteria are undesirable. For hygiene--which technically is "the science and health of preventing disease," they wash a few times daily with hot soapy water. Too much washing isn't good for our skin. It is ironic that the very thing people are using to protect them from disease (soap) is causing skin to become diseased. Try using just Cetaphil or yogurt or honey (my favorite) to cleanse the skin instead, and I don't care how much a fancy cream is, nothing is better than the one God gave you.

Preservation

People are beginning to realize that getting rid of all the bacteria and oils on their skin isn't good, and these are some of the reasons why:

Washing your hands with cold water will help preserve your natural oils.

Your skin is supposed to be slightly acidic, and soap removes this very important acid mantle because it is alkaline. Even water that is piped in from water companies is alkaline; it has to be, because acidic water will corrode plumbing. The slight acidity of the skin protects us from bacteria, fungi, and other microorganisms. Inquire with companies about the pH of the soap you are using, because there are soaps out there that won't destroy the acid mantle.

It's the good bacteria that fight bad bacteria. Let's not leave our skin without any ammunition.

Terribly dry skin can't handle soap or even water, because both are cleansers and remove the acid mantle and natural oils.

To compensate for natural oils washed away, people put creams and oils on their skin. Putting a lot of things on the skin is not good, because creams and lotions can have a drying effect, and long term use of oils encourages the skin to produce less natural oils.

Barrier Function

Calcium significantly helps regulate the barrier function of the skin, and topical red palm oil and sunflower oil also help repair the skin's barrier function. Here's an article from NIH about regarding topical oils and the skin's barrier function. Read the underlined portion of the article that says:

> *"A single application of sunflower seed oil significantly accelerated skin barrier recovery within 1 h; the effect was sustained 5 h after application. In contrast, the other vegetable oils tested (mustard, olive and soybean oils) all significantly delayed recovery of barrier function."*

Note the internal benefits of olive oil in the Free Radical section.

Impact of topical Oils on the Skin Barrier: Possible Implications for Neonatal Health in Developing Countries. Department of International Health, Bloomberg School of Public Health, the Johns Hopkins Medical Institutions, Baltimore, Maryland, USA:

Topical therapy to enhance skin barrier function may be a simple, low-cost, effective strategy to improve outcome of preterm infants with a developmentally compromised epidermal barrier, as lipid constituents of topical products may act as a mechanical barrier and augment synthesis of barrier lipids. Natural oils are applied topically as part of a traditional oil massage to neonates in many developing countries. We sought to identify inexpensive, safe, vegetable oils available in developing countries that improved epidermal barrier function. The impact of oils on mouse epidermal barrier function (rate of transepidermal water loss over time following acute barrier disruption by tape-stripping) and ultra structure was determined. A single application of sunflower seed oil significantly accelerated skin barrier recovery within 1 h; the effect was sustained 5 h after application. In contrast, the other vegetable oils tested (mustard, olive and soybean oils) all significantly delayed recovery of barrier function compared with control- or Aquaphor-treated skin. Twice-daily applications of mustard oil for 7 d resulted in sustained delay of barrier recovery. Moreover, adverse ultra structural changes were seen under transmission electron microscopy in keratin intermediate filament, mitochondrial, nuclear, and nuclear envelope structure following a single application of mustard oil. Conclusion: Our data suggest that topical application of linoleate-enriched oil such as sunflower seed oil might enhance skin barrier function and improve outcome in neonates with compromised barrier function. Mustard oil, used routinely in newborn care throughout South Asia, has toxic effects on the epidermal barrier that warrant further investigation.

PMID: 12113324 [PubMed - indexed for MEDLINE]

Quantitative Analysis of Stratum Corneum Lipids in Xerosis and Asteatotic Eczema. Akimoto K, Yoshikawa N, Higaki Y, Awashima M, Imokawa G. Department of Dermatology, Tokyo

Women's Medical College, Japan.

Sphingolipids, a major constituent of intercellular lipids, are an important determinant for both water-holding and permeability barrier function in the stratum corneum. To assess the pathogenic role of sphingolipids in the stratum corneum of dry skin disorders such as xerosis and asteatotic eczema in leg skin, ceramides were quantified by thin layer chromatography after n-hexane/ethanol extraction of resin-stripped stratum corneum and evaluated as micrograms/mg stratum corneum. In healthy leg skin (n = 49), there was age-related decline in the total ceramide, whereas xerosis (n = 25) and asteatotic eczema (n = 16) suffering significantly reduced water-holding properties, exhibited no definite decrease, rather slight increase in ceramide quantity with the same composition of each individual ceramide as compared to healthy age-matched controls. These data indicate that the seemingly elevated level of ceramide is an artificial effect due to inflammatory processes which result from susceptibility to dryness. Analysis of sebum-derived lipids present in the stratum corneum revealed that there was a significant decline in free fatty acids in xerosis and asteatotic eczema as compared to age-matched healthy controls, and a similar decline in triglycerides in the above three groups when compared to younger controls. Although the observed decrease in the stratum corneum lipids may well explain the high incidence of winter dry skin in older people, the progression toward asteatotic eczema can not be accompanied solely by a decrease in ceramide quantity, suggesting that the evolution of xerotic skin is associated with other moisturizing factors and/or environmental stimuli.

PMID: 8482746 [PubMed - indexed for MEDLINE]

Also see: research about eczema and the barrier function.

External Bacteria

The acid mantle is a protective film formed by the skin. It inhibits the growth of bacteria, fungi, and other microorganisms on the skin's surface. Thus, it is very important to have proper pH on the skin, and you can read more about that in the Acid Mantle section. It has bee noted that people with eczema have too much staphylococcus aureus on their skin, but garlic and salt (FSTR) and honey according to the NIH and the American Academy of Anti-Aging Medicine (especially Manuka honey), and sunflower oil, silver clothing and olive leaf extract are some effective treatments against staphylococcus. Note: vinegar is only slightly effective.

Bacterial and fungal infections can cause some forms of eczema. With this in mind, inflammation is a process which fights infection. So, steroids (which are anti-inflammatory) may worsen the skin condition if it is caused by bacteria or fungus. (See also the Fungus section.) Neomycin Warning: Please note the Antibiotic Ointment Allergy section.

Fungus

Eczema can be a symptom of a systemic candida yeast infection.

"In studies on the pathogenic mechanisms for atopic eczema, we have found that the yeast, Pityrosporum orbiculare, which is normally present on the skin, can act as an allergen." Pityrosporum is a lipophilic yeast form of Malassezia furfur.

Division of Bacterial and Mycotic Diseases. "Persons at high risk for opportunistic fungal infections are those who have undergone ... long-term treatment with corticosteroid or antibacterial drugs."

Recent evidence suggests that the more severe dandruff associated with seborrheic dermatitis may be caused by an overabundance of Pityrosporum ovale, a yeast-like organism found on healthy scalp in low numbers. With the increased scaling and oiliness of seborrheic dermatitis, these yeast organisms thrive and multiply, aggravating inflammation and scaling.

Grapefruit Seed Extract

Effective against staph which is commonly associated with eczema and can be used both internally and externally. I buy mine from the health food store for $10-$20 depending on the size, and it seems to last forever. Teenagers use it instead of soap as a face wash to help with acne, too.

Herbs

There are herbs that can be helpful. See Herbs section.

Vinegar

We know that vinegar has anti-fungal properties. Just 1/4 cup of vinegar in a bathtub filled with water brought down the pH from 9 to below 6. So a splash in the bath may be helpful not only in lowering the pH of highly-alkaline waters, but it can also help fight fungus. Vinegar is not recommended internally if there is a problem with candida.

Garlic and Olive Oil

Garlic helps to fight and prevent the growth of Candida (yeast) and is an effective anti-fungal agent protecting against candidiasis and athlete's foot.

From: Candida Albecans and Multiple Chemical Sensitivities Garlic and olive oil are anti-fungals.

Tea Tree Oil

Some extensive actions of Tea Tree Oil, aka melaluca, include anti-infectious, antiviral, bactericidal, fungicidal.

Antibiotic Ointments

You can start out by reading this: Allergy to Neomycin.

In February 2003 I got a small patch of eczema on my wrist. I attributed it to stress and eating a lot of gluten. Well, to treat the small patch of eczema, I put just a little bit of triple antibiotic ointment. Within a week ... my hands, forearms and face were covered in eczema. Eyes swollen, my skin looked like it had a chemical burn with allergic-looking red bumps, then it would get scaly, dry and itch. I experienced a major eczema outbreak. I didn't realize that I did it to myself until I read in the above link that 30% of people with eczema are allergic to Neomycin, which is an ingredient in triple antibiotic ointments.

Irritant Dermatitis vs. Allergic Contact Dermatitis

Contact dermatitis is divided into two classes: irritant dermatitis and allergic contact dermatitis. Irritant dermatitis is injury due to a non-allergic reaction from direct contact of an irritating substance with the skin such as alkalis and acids. Neomycin, benzocaine and diphenhydramine hydrochloride preparations are topical medications that most commonly cause allergic contact dermatitis.

Neomycin Allergy

Neomycin is usually combined with polymixin B sulfate and bacitracin zinc in over-the-counter antibiotic ointments. Neomycin skin sensitivity was first reported in 1952 by Baer and Ludwig, and contact dermatitis due to Neomycin is most commonly seen in people with atopy, but nonatopic patients are also vulnerable. Allergic contact dermatitis is estimated at 30% in patients with prolonged neomycin exposure (e.g., those with stasis dermatitis).

The AAD warns: neomycin is a common allergen found in both prescription and non-prescription topical antibiotic creams, ointments, lotions, ear drops and eye drops. It is also used in combination with other topical antibiotics, topical steroids and in first aid creams. Neosporin, triple antibiotic creams and ointments contain neomycin. People who are allergic to neomycin and treat their cuts, abrasions, rashes, and poison ivy dermatitis with over-the-counter creams containing neomycin, frequently develop neomycin induced dermatitis.

What to Use Instead

Some people use Polysporin instead which doesn't have neomycin. From dermadoctor.com, apply polysporin ointment into the splits twice a day. Do not use any topical antibiotic ointment that contains neomycin which is a notorious skin sensitizer and cause of contact dermatitis. Red Palm Oil also helps fight infection and so does olive leaf extract.

Inflammation

Inflammation comes in cycles, and once the cycle is broken the inflammation will subside. From a brochure by NEASE:

> *"We know that AD is a disease of inflamed skin. That inflammation is a result of various cells coming into the skin and causing itching, redness and swelling. Those cells come from the person's bone marrow, then they travel through the blood stream to the target tissues: the skin in AD, the nose in hay fever, the lungs in asthma. Something makes these cells over-react. They generate too much inflammation and they don't stop. Maybe that's the cause of the disease--cells that create too much damage when they turn on and they don't turn off the way they should. We don't know the reason for the defective "on/off switch." We can only try to control AD by preventing the "on" trigger. Things that turn "on" the switch are called trigger factors."*

I don't entirely agree with that. Sometimes the body knows better than we do. Ya think? (lol) There can be good reasons for inflammation; and, instead of just suppressing it, we might need to look at and then deal with the underlying cause which might be a bacterial infection. I understand the immune system has memory, and glyconutrients are helpful with that. Regarding the drug Protopic (tacrolimus), which is an immunosuppressant, see the Fungus section for some interesting insight. Also, if you have had problems with Protopic and Elidel with regards to cancer, see: Larry M. Roth, PA

See, also, this Harvard article entitled, "What you eat can fuel or cool inflammation."

Corticosteroids

New research says most cases of eczema (two-thirds) is from a defective barrier function and from skin that is too thin, but the #1 prescribed medicines is hydrocortisone which thins the skin.

From <u>Croatian Medical Journal</u>, "Conclusion. Previous long-term topical treatment resulted in allergic contact dermatitis in most of the patients, and to a lesser extent in irritant contact dermatitis or a combination of seborrheic dermatitis and rosaceiform dermatitis. The data stress the importance of avoiding long-term topical treatment with corticosteroids, antibiotics and aggressive agents."

Tapering off should be done slowly or the condition can flare up. I'll tell you how I tapered off: First, I started using them only when my skin was soaking wet with water, because that diluted it. Then, I used less and less of it each time I applied. Then, I skipped applications. Then, I skipped days. Within a short time, I had weaned myself off of the external steroids. Ask your physician how you should do it.

Please note: Clearly I am not saying never use corticosteroids, because they can be helpful sometimes. I would like to emphasize, though, that there are many things you can be doing to lessen your dependence upon them and even come to a point where you don't ever need them. When using corticosteroids, remember that cortisone creams tend to have a drying effect and for this reason are better for weepy eczema, and ointments are better for dry eczema.

Corticosteroids and What Happened to Me

When traditional/western medicine failed me, I didn't get better until I went the naturopathic/holistic way. However, after being well for a few years, I was overexposed to harmful chemicals at school for months on end and experienced a breakout. For one year after that I tried so many natural remedies to get better, but it just seemed like the more I tried and experimented with natural remedies, the worse I got. My skin was in such a hypersensitive state that everything irritated it … even water. I couldn't get better. I was stuck.

Later, I learned that the reason I couldn't clear up the eczema the naturopathic way during that year was because of taking a medicine, so make sure you check out the list of drugs to see if you're taking something that might be causing you to have a rash: Drugs that Cause Rashes.

Finally, I went back to a dermatologist for testing thinking it was maybe a bacterial infection or something. What happened, though, was that although internal modifications are great and helpful and are what it took to get me well and keep me well the first time around after suffering for a couple of decades, it was a medicine I was taking for stress and things I was putting on my skin that were irritating it this time around. My skin was so hypersensitive that it couldn't tolerate anything at all.

The dermatologist instructed me to use pure mineral oil topically after a 10 minute warm soak in the bathtub. Please note that your skin will absorb water for the first 10 minutes, but after 10 minutes the water will begin to dry out your skin (it'll shrivel up and wash away your natural oils). Mineral oil is found in the laxative section at the drugstore. He said there is only one thing he knows of that would lubricate the skin and not cause an allergic reaction: mineral oil, because it's inert. He was right. It didn't burn me or cause me to itch like all the natural oils did, and God knows I tried everything under the sun I could think of. Remember also that every company for eczema out there gave me stuff for free to try because of my www.eczema.net web site, but I didn't find one single product to help me ... not one. That's why I don't have any for sale on my site. Sure mineral oil is an occlusive barrier and smother the skin with long term use; but, that's exactly what we need when the skin is messed up until it can heal over. It's a good band-aid. It was the only skin band-aid I knew of that wouldn't cause a reaction on hypersensitive skin. Vaseline caused me to break out.

He also gave me prescriptions that dealt with the inflammation: a) on the face: hydrocortisone ointment 2.5%; and, b) on the rest of my body alternate or mix together (however I wanted) but to apply more than generously even up to 100 times a day to keep the skin moist: **Betamethasone Valerate Cream 0.1% and Betamethasone Valerate Ointment 0.1%**. This is important: applying a lot of this medium strength cortisone on the skin (even "up to 10 times daily," he said) isn't at all like taking them internally in terms of potential negative side effects. In other words putting that medium strength steroid on the skin many times daily is much safer than taking them internally. So there you go, taking dangerous levels of internal steroids didn't help me at all; but, applying that medium strength steroid onto the skin itself very generously did. I wonder why in the world I had never been instructed to do that before in all my years of suffering. Appling non-prescription steroids topically three to four times daily was definitely not enough to stop the cycle of inflammation that I was experiencing from the extreme chemical damage done to my skin. As a matter of fact, I think my skin gets worse using hydrocortisone; but, applying Betamethasone Valerate generously always hits the reset button in my case. I don't believe in living off of cortisones, but I do believe in using them sometimes. Why doctors prescribe the dangerous internal steroids before using the external steroids generously is beyond me.

The last tricky part came after my skin had calmed down, the rash was gone, and I still needed to lubricate. Somehow that magical mineral oil that did wonders for my skin later seemed to make my skin lifeless. It was great for helping me heal up, but for the long term it was smothering my skin. Now that the skin is under control, though, I can use other lighter all natural products and not have the allergic reaction because my skin is now in a calmer state. I actually use Burt's Bees milk and honey lotion regularly. Since adding calcium to my diet, though, my skin doesn't even get too dry anymore except a little after I take a shower.

Honey is also a potent anti-inflammatory, antimicrobial, has an acid pH, helps keep the moisture in, causes no tissue damage, significantly increases production of collagen and has no negative side effects when used topically (allergy to honey is rare). Read this honey link, and you will begin to see why honey worked better for me than even cortisones. Remember, though, don't give honey internally to infants.

Hopefully the knowledge in this book will help bring you to a place where you don't need to live off steroids like I did my first 15 years of suffering. They didn't even help me, but that's all

I knew and trusted in with western medicine. On the other hand, don't be so rigid that you refuse to use the cortisones under any circumstances. I trust, though, we'll bring you to the point where you won't have to use them all.

Ingredients

This was a tricky subject. I tried to bring logic into the debate of why questionable ingredients are found in products that can be helpful. In 1996 I discovered that if I avoided lanolin, my skin was better. It made sense because wool made me feel itchy and lanolin comes from wool. Some people told me that lanolin doesn't bother their eczema, but more people told me that it does. Different things can affect different people differently because we are biochemically different.

Cetyl alcohol, propylene glycol, glycerin, sodium laureth sulfate, sodium lauryl sulfate, parabens, fragrances, petroleum products, mineral oils and list the goes on have come up as being bad ingredients. I have cautioned people about some of the above ingredients; but, I had to figure out why formulators of dermatological products use some of the above-listed ingredients and why their products have helped people.

Let's quickly just look at couple of ingredients to give you a general picture. Cetyl alcohol is a fatty acid alcohol and not a drying alcohol like methyl alcohol (rubbing alcohol) or ethyl alcohol (drinking alcohol). Propylene glycol, used as a preservative and humectant, is used in a very small amount in some skin products. Formulators agree that when used in large amounts it is an anti-freeze. Basic chemistry shows us that chemicals used at varying strengths have different chemical reactions. If propylene glycol is horrible in small quantities, then why haven't formulators been banned from using it, and why do biochemists feel comfortable using it? Sometimes chemicals can be used in very small quantities and formulated with other chemicals which can offset the negatives of questionable chemicals.

The analogy that comes to my mind is one that has to do with hydrochloric acid. We need a small amount in our stomach to digest food (we can become ill from the lack of it); but, if we go drinking lots of it, it's a killer. Similarly, our skin has a healthy acid mantle, but if we go pouring lots of acid on the skin, it'll burn us. A little acid with a lot of water is a lot different than a lot of acid with a little water.

I'm not trying to whitewash anything; rather, I am trying to bring logic into why biochemists concerned about things like cortisone and detergents who are educated and earnestly trying to develop products that will help skin will use some chemicals that have been blacklisted. I believe that the proportion of chemicals is of utmost importance and that varying sensitivities and proportions of chemicals play a larger role than would appear on the surface. It's the only logical explanation why questionable ingredients are found in products that have been helpful.

In my experience, using pure vaseline (white petrolatum) on my skin made me feel itchy. But, there are products with those ingredients that have helped me. Things that produce a lot of suds bother my skin. Sodium laureth sulfate and sodium lauryl sulfate help form suds. But, there are products designed for eczema that have those ingredients in them and have helped people with eczema. Regarding fragrance, one manufacturer wrote saying that they use the least reactive fragrance that is available. They also wrote that parabens are the least reactive of the available preservatives and said that the sensitivity rate of their products is less than 1%.

So, the bottom line must be what are the proportions of the chemicals, how do they interact with the other chemicals in the product, and what are the results of the products being used on our skin as we biochemically differ. It is my experience that only small amounts of products should be used, and remember: preservation of your natural oil is best.

Cleansers

Remember: even running water has cleansing action, and sometimes just a good rinse is all that is warranted--you only need something other than water under the arms, the groin and the soles of the feet. To preserve natural oils, use warm (not hot) water and rinse with cool water. Restoring and maintaining the proper pH of your acid mantle is important. I use plain yogurt (pH of 4.2) to cleanse the skin. If there is an infection, an antibacterial cleanser may be needed, but restore the good bacteria on the skin with yogurt or probiotics. The cleanser Cetaphil (you can get the generic brand) is pretty gentle on the skin.

At one point, I liked using distilled water to rinse my hands when they were inflamed, because the water coming out of my tap had a pH of 9, and that was too high. Plus, it's chlorinated and that may affect the good bacteria. See the Acid Mantle section.

Here's a very interesting article on the pH of different soaps and their effects on the skin.

Water

I was wondering what was used for thousands of years before soap was invented, so I did an electronic search in the Bible for the word "wash." The phrase "wash with water" came up repetitively. It is the mechanics of running water that washes away dirt, and water is a file solvent for salt.

pH of Water

To learn why pH is important, please visit the <u>Acid Mantle</u> section. In a nutshell, we want products with a pH of 4.5 to 6.5 on the skin. It's important, because alkaline water and products can also cause drying of the skin.

Water piped in from water companies is alkaline to preserve plumbing and to prevent lead and copper from seeping out of pipes (acidic water corrodes plumbing). The water being piped into my home comes in at a pH of 9. If your water is highly alkaline, adding a splash of apple cider vinegar which is acidic to the bath can help combat the problem of dry skin (restoring acidity). I use a skin toner to restore the proper pH on my face. Well water tends to be acidic. If it's too acidic, adding some baking soda will raise the pH. Distilled water has a pH of between 5.6 and 7.

Testing pH

If you experiment with the pH of your water, get a pH test kit. They are not expensive, and you can get them from your local pool store. Also, pool stores will test your water for you. I don't think they'll charge you. Further, you can ask your water companies to come and test the pH level of the water in your homes.

Jacuzzi to Lower pH

If you have a jacuzzi, turning it on and bubbling air through the water will lower the pH of the water so that it is close to 7 (neutral) by dissolving some extra carbon dioxide in it. (Thank you Physics Professor, Dr. Bloomfield.)

Epsom Salt (Magnesium Sulfate)

Epsom salt is hydrated magnesium sulfate (about 10 percent magnesium and 13 percent sulfur). It will lower the pH of the water in the bath and is especially useful in treating wounds and widespread eruptions of the skin, removing crusts, scales and relieving inflammation and itching; and it can help take the sting out of insect bites. It didn't sting or burn my skin like salty ocean water did when the skin was raw. (2 cups of epsom salt in a warm bath.)

Epsom salt is also used to make wet dressings. It helps drain swollen tissues, boils, infection and will draw toxins and splinters out of the skin. (2 cups of epsom salt in 2 cups of hot water to make a compress; apply as a wet dressing with a towel.)

Bath Water

See, also, the <u>Bath</u> section to learn why people with dry skin and eczema might consider taking 10 minutes baths.

Thermal Suits and Wet Wraps/Evaporation Method

Below is all about the evaporation or wet wrap method; but, before you do that and get cold, totally try the Thermal Suit method, because it's the only thing I do. I don't have to use lotions or wet wraps anymore. You can pick one up at Job Lot for about $10 or at sporting goods store like Dick's. It's like wearing a light weight jogging suit made of vinyl. I put it on over my clothes and wear it around all day (out shopping and everything). It's great, because I don't have to use lotions after I shower, I never feel cold anymore, and when I take my suit off at night, my clothes are very, very damp, so I know I have trapped my moisture in without using lotions or creams.

Now, about the famous wet wrap method:

From How Things Work with Louis A. Bloomfield, Professor of Physics, The University of Virginia). My question and his answer.

Q. How is the skin better hydrated by vapor as opposed to liquid water? Wrapping yourself in a damp sheet is more effective at treating the dryness of eczema than taking a bath. -- Christina Nevada

A. " When your skin is immersed in pure water, the only molecules that ever collide with its surface are water molecules. That might seem to be the ideal situation for keeping skin moist, however such immersion can have other unintended consequences. First, any water soluble atoms, molecules, and ions that can move to the surface of your skin will dissolve away in the surrounding water and you'll never see them again. Second, any water soluble atoms, molecules, and ions that can't move to the surface of your skin will draw water into your skin by way of osmosis--the pure water will flow into your skin cells in an attempted to dilute the dissolved particles inside those cells. After a relatively short time, the cells of your skin will contain many more water molecules than before and your skin will look all wrinkly. This flow of water soluble materials out of your skin and water into your skin may not be so wonderful for your eczema."

"When you wrap yourself in a wet cloth, you are ensuring that the relative humidity near the surface of your skin will be close to 100%. Air molecules will still be present around your skin but now there will be essentially no net transfer of water between your skin and the surrounding air--water molecules will leave your skin for the air at roughly the same rate as water molecules return to your skin from the air. In effect, you are stopping evaporation from your skin and very little else. Stopping evaporation from your skin will also cause it to accumulate moisture, but this time the new moisture will come from within your body. Water molecules that would have left your skin had it been surrounded by dry air are now staying in your skin, where they add to the moisture in your skin. Overall, your skin will contain more water but it will not have lost as many water soluble chemicals and it will not have water driven into it by osmotic pressure. It may be this more gentle moisturizing effect that makes wrapping yourself in a damp sheet more pleasant for your eczema than immersing yourself in water."

Key in on the word "vapor". Just laying damp sheets over the skin is all you really have to do. I learned about it from Yale Dermatology, and it was effective enough to break the cycle of my inflammation that was biopsied three times by other doctors. When they told me to lay damp sheets on the skin, I responded that it was probably the hydration that was helpful. In answer to that comment, the dermatologist told me that evaporation breaks down skin inflammation. That's why I began to call it the Evaporation Method instead of just wet wrapping.

Evaporation has two descriptions: 1) to draw moisture from; and 2) the conversion of water into vapor. Zoom in on the second description, and let's correlate it with wet wrap therapy. Why use a wet wrap instead of just a bath? Liquid water is not as effective in hydrating skin as water vapor. Just like water evaporates out of our skin, water vapor can hydrate the skin. Baths didn't help me; only when the wetness began to evaporate out of the sheet did I see and feel improvement. Remember, hydration of the skin will result in reduced inflammation.

Feedback

"I don't think I can thank you enough for the help you gave me. I have eczema all over my body. The only thing the doctors could say is steroids shots to clear me up. It has been 3 days now since I have been using the wet wraps, and I am almost cleared up. THANK YOU, THANK YOU. My doctor never heard of it. Keep spreading the information."

"Thank you for your eczema relief remedy. Our son who is now 1 year old has been battling eczema his whole life. We have tried everything! .... We will try your water bath sheet therapy! Thank you so much for your helpful hint." Later, she wrote back with this: *"Our son's eczema has really cleared up! We have been using Aveeno skin cleanser instead of soap and shampoo for him."*

"I woke up with a couple of spots. Did the first half hour evaporation, and that's all it took. It's evening now, and I was going to do another half hour, but there's nothing there. Amazing!!!!! Thank you!" "Try the evaporation trick ..., it seems to curb the intense itching sensation."

"The evaporation thing works wonders, and even if I am not "cured" my skin is getting better, not worse. I will continue to try Chinese herbs (as I can afford it!) and some other alternative things, but at least this is manageable now."

This is why I believe that we need to take this simple knowledge and give it the stardom it deserves. Before I explain how I used evaporation, it's important to share with you something another person wrote:

"I tried the evaporation method and have mixed feelings. I felt better at the start--the inflammation went down; but, it came back with a vengeance the next day."

I responded to her this way ... Since the evaporation method helped the inflammation subside, I should ask what you did later that might be causing the flare-ups. Evaporation can break the cycle of inflammation, but it may return unless the irritant is avoided. For, something as simple as a lotion with lanolin might be causing the flare-ups.

Some Ways to Use Wet Wraps

Because water evaporates out of a sheet/pillow case quickly, dampen it in WARM water, quickly squeeze out the excess water (it shouldn't be dripping wet), and then lay it over the inflammation until the skin feels better. I say warm water because it feels better, and it will get cold soon enough anyway. Try using a white 100% cotton sheet or pillow case. If you can avoid 50% cotton & 50% polyester, it might be helpful because some polyester blends make me feel itchy. Rewet it every 15 minutes or so. The itchiness should begin to subside within 5 minutes. Half an hour to an hour can make a noticeable difference. When the eczema was out of control, I used wet wraps three times daily.

Wrap yourself up in the damp sheet, and lounge around in it if it's warm enough. I realize this is going to make you feel chilled. So, you can go ahead and wrap a blanket around yourself, too. You can sleep with damp pillow cases covering the areas of inflammation.

Make cover-ups from pillow cases for children.

If it's too cold to do that, you can also sit in a bathtub with just enough WARM water to make you comfortable. Then, put the damp sheet on the inflammation. Keep warming the water and draining the cooled water so you don't get too cold. Remember, as the water evaporates out of the sheet, you will feel better.

Try using a cotton dress shirt.

Put your arms in a damp pillow case while you watch TV.

One night I woke up with my back feeling hot, sweaty and itchy with a patchy raised rash (eczema). I got a pillow case, dampened it with warm water, squeezed out the excess water, took it back to bed, laid down on my stomach, put the pillow case on my back, covered up with my blanket, the itch subsided after a couple of minutes, I fell asleep like that; and, when I woke up, the inflammation had subsided. This is a pattern. I can depend on it for reliable help.

A student e-mailed me that he made a mask from a pillow case so that he could study while using evaporation.

Try buying 100% cotton light weight pajamas and use them instead of sheets. Then, maybe put another pair of those pajamas on top so that it's not too cold.

Don't use towels to dry your body after taking a shower;

just brush away the water with your hands to preserve your natural oils.

Repetitive splashing of very cold water on your skin should rinse off any irritant and help the itch subside.

Dry Skin with Wet Wraps

Whatever way of using wet wraps, if your skin feels tight, putting on an irritant-free moisturizer while the skin is still wet with water droplets may be helpful.

Baths

NaPCA

Skin will absorb water for the first 10 minutes; then, after skin is immersed in water for longer than that, the primary humectant in human skin (NaPCA) migrates into the bath water. This is why the skin feels tight after getting out of the bath. The bath water, if alkaline, will also dry the skin.

Health Dept. Recommendations

Connecticut State Health Officials recommend a lukewarm shower once every 4 days for the general public. They realize that taking too many baths and showers damages the skin. My pediatrician also recommends the same for all children. Preservation of natural oils is key in eczema management. This single aspect of care can go far in helping people with eczema.

Soap Residue

Many pediatricians say we do not need to use any cleansers on our children's skin other than water. Water is a cleanser. Huggies Natural Care Unscented Alcohol-Free Baby Wipes (lanolin-free) can be used in between shower days to cleanse the bottom and under the arms, but I'm wonder if some skin is reacting to it. Try using yogurt instead and rinse it off. The Acid Mantle section describes why people with eczema should not use regular soap.

Bacterial and Fungal Infections

Please also refer to the Bacteria section, because infection can be a factor behind skin rashes. This is why some doctors prescribe baths with a small amount of bleach.

Showering

State Health Officials recommend a lukewarm shower once every 4 days (with normal activity). My pediatrician also recommends the same. Many pediatricians say we **do not** need to use any cleansers on our children's skin other than water (unless they been playing in sandboxes and such). In between those days, a wet wash cloth can be used to cleanse under the arms and the bottom as needed with something gentle like Cetaphil. I just use plain water or plain yogurt. Here's a very interesting article on the pH of different soaps and their effects on the skin.

Preservation of your natural oils is key in eczema management. This single aspect of care will go far in helping people with eczema. Continued use of hot soapy water every day from head to toe destroys the hydrolipid film and acid mantle. Without them, the skin is going to have a tough time staying healthy. Remember, though, that if there's an underlying bacterial infection, that needs to be addressed. Probiotics are helpful.

Now that I'm better, I can shower pretty much as I want to; but, it was hard showering when I was sick with eczema, because even the water burned my skin.

See, also, the Bath section.

Shampooing

The Inflamed Scalp

When I first got eczema on my scalp, I just kept shampooing it every day to get rid of the flaking. My scalp became very red, inflamed and terribly itchy. As it worsened, I used shampoos for scalp problems like Nizoral and T-Gel. My scalp became even more inflamed. It got so bad that I lost half of my hair.

How I Recovered

Since shampooing wasn't helping, I decided to apply the theory that "soap can hurt damaged skin", and I began the backward habit of just using water to wash my hair for four days. Steadily, the inflammation and flaking subsided. I also used apple cider vinegar and a tiny bit of jojoba oil on the scalp while I was "recovering from shampoo damage" and combating any possible fungus. Later, I discovered yogurt was the best thing to use. See, also, the Bacteria section, because using Sea Breeze or another astringent or toner can also be helpful like vinegar in this regard.

pH of Hair Products is Very Important

When we don't use pH balanced products on the hair, the alkaline shampoos can mess up our scalp ... and our hair, because it's the acidic pH that makes the cuticle of the hair lay flat making hair healthier and shinier. Alkaline hair products not only destroy our natural acid mantle on our scalp which is supposed to protect us from bacteria and fungus, but they also open the cuticle of the hair and damages hair. So, when you buy hair products, go to a salon or a beauty supply store and ask them for hair products that are acidic and not alkaline. You can also search for "acidic pH hair products" on the Net. Yogurt has a pH of 4.2.

Shampooing Habits

When I was recovering, I washed my hair just every 4th day. In between those days, I rinsed any excess salt, dust or oils out of the hair with warm water and then rinsed with cool water. If my scalp ever gets itchy, I use apple cider vinegar or Sea Breeze and it stops the itch and prevents the scalp from going crazy like it did before. A tablespoon of Sea Breeze in a cup and a half of water as a final rinse is also helpful. Generally, you can rinse it every day and use conditioner ... just don't use shampoo every day (once or twice a week is much better for you).

I didn't get my whole body wet when washing my hair. Just leaned over the side of the bathtub and washed my hair that way. That avoided getting suds over the rest of my skin. Using plastic gloves and a long handled back brush to wash your hair and your children's hair will spare your hands as well.

Rinse conditioners with out with cold (not warm) water.

Chemicals in Shampoos

The chemicals sodium laureth/lauryl sulfate can irritate sensitive skin. These chemicals help form suds.

The Ingredients section may also help clear up some issues about chemicals.

Jojoba Oil

Jojoba oil is helpful. You can find the oil in your local health food stores.

Hair Loss

I lost more than half of the thickness of my beautiful, healthy, treasured long hair. It fell out by the strand in the shower, and I would find it on my pillow in the morning. So sad it was. I gave it a blunt shoulder length cut to make it look thicker.

I tried the shampoos for eczema, but they all made my scalp more inflamed. It was red and oh so very, very itchy. I think that scratching it contributed to the hair loss like an animal gets bald patches from scratching, but I know it fell from the panic attacks, too.

I'll tell you what saved me, it was using apple cider vinegar externally and a little bit of jojoba oil. I've since learned that apple cider vinegar and sage tea as a rinse will help hair grow. I started soaking my scalp with the vinegar and left it on for one hour. Then I rinsed it out and put a little bit of jojoba oil where it felt dry. What an immediate improvement. It put all that other stuff I tried to shame. Taking Biotin also helps stop hair from falling out. Using yogurt as a shampoo can be helpful. The pH is 4.2 (not alkaline).

So, whenever my scalp feels a little itchy (not much at all any more), I take a water bottle filled with vinegar and squirt some on my scalp. Next, I get a white kitchen trash bag and put my hair in it like a shower cap and then wrap a towel around my head so the excess vinegar won't drip down and burn my forehead. Doing that once a week stops the problem from coming back. It helps a lot to kill and control the itch, too. This method is very helpful to kill the itch anywhere that hair grows.

Sea Breeze astringent can also be helpful. (See the Bacteria section) and note the Fungus section, because dandruff is caused by a fungus. This is why vinegar is helpful. Using a toner on the eyebrows will help with the flaking.

CAUTION: Vinegar will sting damaged skin a lot. Just start drop by drop diluted with water to see if it stings too much; and, if it's okay, increase to full strength.

pH of Hair Products is Very Important

When we don't use pH balanced products on the hair, the alkaline shampoos can mess up our scalp ... and our hair, because it's the acidic pH that makes the cuticle of the hair lay flat making hair healthier and shinier. Alkaline hair products not only destroy our natural acid mantle on our scalp which is supposed to protect us from bacteria and fungus, but they also open the cuticle of the hair and damages hair. So, when you buy hair products, go to a salon or a beauty supply store and ask them for hair products that are acidic and not alkaline. You can also search for "acidic pH hair products" on the Net.

Eyebrow Loss

Try using an acidic toner like Sea Breeze liberally ... and maybe even a topical antibiotic like Polysporin, since it could be a bacterial issue.

Helpful Supplements

Biotin, essential fatty acids, B vitamins, vitamin E, zinc, vitamin A, vitamin C and lecithin are helpful. Lack of stomach acid contributes to hair loss. Regarding herbs, chaparral or thyme may be used as a hair rinse. Taking dandelion, goldenseal and red clover can also be helpful.

Circulation and Hair Nutrition

Massaging the scalp daily (not scratching it though) and lying angled down to increase circulation and blood flow to the scalp can also encourage hair growth, and taking hair vitamins is key.

Creams and Lotions & Oils and Ointments

Creams and lotions can sometimes have a drying effect. Creams can be helpful for drying weepy eczema, and oils and ointments are better for dry eczema. Please note that just as drying agents used on the skin for acne can encourage the skin to produce more oil, overuse of oils on the skin can discourage the skin from producing natural oils. Moderation is good.

Although mineral oil can suffocate the skin with long term use, for short term use while the skin needs a band-aid, it's one thing I know of that won't aggravate sensitive skin, because it's inert. You'll find it in the laxative section at the stores. However, sunflower oil improves the barrier function of the skin. However, to get something on the skin that has benefit action, check out the benefits of Red Palm Oil.

Internal Help

Consume good fats like flax and olive oil to moisturize from within. To help regulate the sweat and oil glands, get enough biotin, zinc and water. Hyaluronic acid is needed to cushion and lubricate joints, eyes, skin and heart valves. See Calcium.

My Motto

The less you over wash your skin, the less you'll dry it out. The less you dry it out, the less you need to put on it. The less you put on, the less you aggravate it, and putting a lot of anything on the skin can make it itchy. Please also see The Proper Perspective Section.

Developing sensitivities can be a concern for some people. I've heard people say things like, "I've used that product a long time and it can't possibly be aggravating my terrible case of eczema." People develop sensitivities over time. The treatment for chemical sensitivity is avoidance, this decreases the total body burden and allows for the recovery of the overtaxed detoxification system. I like to use a product for a while, switch to something else, and then switch back again. This way the chances of becoming sensitive to products is lessened.

A word of caution ... lanolin can aggravate eczema. Refer to: the Ingredients and Anti-Itch sections.

Occlusive Barriers

With eczema, it has long been the practice to seal in moisture with occlusive barriers like mineral oil, petrolatum, lanolin and beeswax to prevent the skin from drying out. That's a nice thought, but since the skin needs to breathe, it isn't good for it in the long run. Using them as a band-aid until the skin heals is good though. Mineral oil is best, because it is inert and won't cause itching on hypersensitive skin. Occlusive barriers can clog the pores and in the long run lead to unhealthy skin that dries out easily. What we need to do is encourage the skin to maintain proper hydration, and here are some things we can do:

Drink more water because if you don't have enough in your system, your body will pull it from the skin to get what it needs.

Preserve our natural oils: The more we wash off our natural oils with water and cleansers, the less we have.

The more oil we use, the more we encourage our skin to produce less natural oils, but check out the Red Palm Oil link for amazing benefits and read about Sunflower oil.

Make sure you're getting your enzymes to break down fats and essential fatty acids.

Humectants

Humectants are ingredients that act as water attractors by pulling moisture from the air and towards the skin. The only potential problem is that if the air is dry (if humidity is below 66%), they pull moisture out of the skin instead of the air.

Dry Eczema vs. Weepy Eczema

Dry Eczema

Remember that creams and lotions can be drying and that heavy, long term use of oils can cause the skin to produce less natural oils. Soap dries the skin and so does even water.

Preservation of the natural oils is best. I don't use soap much anymore at all; I use cream cleansers but mostly just water. You can even use yogurt to cleanse. Remember also that soap residue in clothes dries the skin, so use less detergent and try double rinsing the clothes. You can even coat the skin with oil before you shower to help protect your oils.

For really dry areas, take some distilled water and moisten a cotton pad. Add just a little mineral oil which is inert or honey or whatever your favorite topical product is and place it on the dry patch with a super size band aid or saran wrap. Leave on overnight. If your skin is so hypersensitive and itchy, go to the Corticosteroids section.

Calcium, drinking enough water, getting your essential fatty acids and enzymes to break down the fats may also be helpful.

Weepy Eczema

Nothing seemed to help the weepy patches of eczema better than zinc oxide ointment. It dried the eczema cuts on my hands (seems like overnight). When my face was having an allergic reaction, zinc oxide ointment took care of stopping the golden drops from oozing out of my face. (My cheeks first became tingly, then bright red and then oozed.) I avoided soap on my cheeks and used cool water and zinc oxide ointment.

Remember, though, that external bacteria and fungus can be a reason for rashes, as was the case with my hands, eyebrows and hair. Using a toner on the skin to restore the proper pH will help fight infections.

Watery, Itchy Blisters

Dermatitis herpetiformis (DH) is a chronic disease of the skin marked by groups of watery, itchy blisters that may resemble pimples or blisters. The ingestion of gluten (from wheat, rye, and barley) triggers an immune system response that deposits a substance, IgA (Immunoglobulin A), under the top layer of skin. IgA is present in affected as well as unaffected skin. DH is an autoimmune gluten intolerance disease linked with celiac disease. With DH, the primary lesion is on the skin, whereas with celiac disease the lesions are in the small intestine. The degree of damage to the small intestine is often less severe or more patchy than those with celiac disease.

Itching

Itch signals are similar to pain signals and occupy the same nerve fibers. Substances like histamine (the amine that causes widening of blood vessels) are set free and irritate nerve fibers in the skin. Why does scratching feel so good? Scratching occupies the nerve fibers and blocks the itch messages being sent to the central nervous system. Healthy, normal scratching can remove the stimulus causing the itching (like a hair) and can sometimes trigger an immune response to remove the cause of the irritation. That's the good news about scratching.

However, with eczema, scratching and rubbing causes thick skin. Abnormally thick skin sends more messages of itch and fuels the Itch/Scratch Cycle. Scratching also causes injury to the skin and direct release of inflammatory mediators that enhance or cause itching themselves. The more people with eczema scratch, the further they cause the inflammation that triggers the itch.

See, also, the Watery, Itchy Blisters section.

Antihistamines: Are They Helpful?

I worked my way up to 20 antihistamines daily; but, even with that dosage, I was still tormented with severe itching.

From: The University of Nottingham

> *The mechanism of itch in atopic eczema is still unknown. Some of the pruritus in atopic eczema may be induced by non-histamine mechanisms such as neuroactive peptides or central mechanisms. Histamine is the most thoroughly studied pruritogenic mediator and was for long assumed to be the unique itch stimulus. Today, a number of other peripheral inflammatory mediators are known to act as pruritogenics, either by acting directly on peripheral nerve endings, or indirectly by releasing endogenous substances that in turn stimulate the nerve endings, for example serotonin, proteases (e.g. kallikrein, papain), peptides (e.g. bradykinin, sekretin) and prostaglandins (e.g. PGE1, PGE2 and PGH2) (Wahlgren, 1991). Histamine is the main itch-provoking substance in urticaria, but the role of histamine in other itching disorders including atopic eczema remains to be defined. It is not understood, why for example erythema, sweating, dry skin or wool elicits itch in patients with AE and to what degree factors other than histamine play a role. Further, it is unclear whether potential beneficial effects of sedating antihistamines are due to their central effects (sedation) alone or due to their peripheral effects. In many tests and management guideline articles (McHenry et al., 1995), it is claimed that sedative antihistamines are more effective than low-sedating antihistamines. This appears to be based on scanty data (Krause & Shuster, 1983). Another issue relating to the use of antihistamines in atopic eczema is that they can only be used for short periods because tolerance to the effects is thought to develop quite quickly (Kemp, 1989). Another area of concern is that antihistamines have been linked with*

behavior disorders such as hyperactivity in children (Calmels et al., 1982). So it is not clear

> *i) if antihistamines are helpful in AE*
> *ii) whether only sedating ones are helpful*
> *iii) how long they are helpful for and*
> *iv) whether they demonstrate undesirable side effects*

From Merck, "Antihistamines are ineffective in suppressing allergic contact dermatitis."

Techniques to Help Curb Itching

If the sky is itching from being dry or from putting things on it that make it itch, try mineral oil since it's inert. Read the Cortisone section for important information.

Course Washcloth: Sometimes you feel itchy because of the uneven skin feeling like little hairs that you need to scratch off. I find that just gently rubbing the skin with a course washcloth smoothes the skin and helps alleviate that externally stimulated itch.

Ice Therapy: Dry eczema should not get wet to preserve the natural oils. Try filling a plastic bottle (such as an empty vitamin bottle) with water and freeze it. It can help block the itch signals and reduce the inflammation. From Ice Therapy, "Ice decreases all of these: swelling, tissue damage, blood clot formation, inflammation, muscle spasms, and pain."

Heat Therapy: Something I noticed that works is heat. If I feel itchy, I take a hot water bottle and leave it on the skin until it hurts a little bit, and then the itch goes away. Watch out, though, because you can get burned. Unfortunately, some people stand under the shower with the water as hot as they can stand it, because it alleviates their itch, so use the hot water bottle instead of that, because it won't dry out the skin. I even used to use a blow dryer to the point of getting burned to try and alleviate the itch, but that left the skin even worse off. Hot water bottles are the best so far. The Itch Stopper works on that same premise, too, heat, only a hot water bottle covers a lot more territory really quick and is much, much cheaper ... and doesn't even require batteries. (lol)

Wet Wraps: Another way to handle the itching is using the Evaporation Method (Wet Wraps).

Vinegar: Apple cider vinegar kills the itch nicely where hair grows. Watch, though, because it can horribly sting broken skin. Dilute it first on broken skin and then work your way up to full strength ... always test small areas first. It killed sunburn itch when nothing else did.

You Can Get Better, Too

My once insane itch that led me to take twenty antihistamines daily is gone. Thank God not everyone with eczema has this extreme itch, otherwise known as pruritus "severe itching." So, I avoided as much as possible touching things that made me itch even more like detergents and acidic foods; and, when I did feel itchy from touching something, I rinsed that part of the skin with cold water and tried not to scratch with my fingernails (used my knuckles instead).

Some people rinse with cool water and then get in front of a fan ... it's very chilly, but can be helpful, too.

For an in-depth article on itching, see: American Family Physician on Pruritis ("Itching").

Scarring

The general rule of thumb is to protect the scar from the sun for the first year so that later it will tan and fade with the rest of the skin. In time, scars will fade. Cuts can be dried up rather quickly with zinc oxide ointment (and it acts like a sunscreen, too).

Regarding bleeding, I learned many years ago from the emergency room that hydrogen peroxide (about .50 a bottle in the grocery store) very easily gets blood out of material. It has never changed the color of the fabric in all the years I've used it on clothing, sheets, blankets and carpeting.

But, I guess the first thing we should think about is why the scarring ... thin skin that tears easily from the use of external steroids and scratching ... I got over it, and I sure think that you can, too.

Clothing

Silver-Coated Textiles in the Therapy of Atopic Eczema

Gauger A. Hipler U.-C., Elsner P (eds): Biofunctional Textiles and the Skin. Curr Probl Dermatol. Basel, Karger, 2006, vol 33, pp 152-164 (DOI: 10.1159/000093942). Medline Abstract (ID 16766887)

Atopic skin is mainly determined by a disrupted skin barrier, resulting in a higher susceptibility to external irritants in affected and nonaffected skin. Apart from many other irritant and allergic influences, skin colonization with Staphylococcus aureus is one of the major factors triggering and maintaining atopic eczema (AE). Adequate textile protection with low irritant potential can be helpful in reducing the exposure to exogenous trigger factors. Until now, cotton fabrics have been the state of the art of recommended textiles for patients with AE. The combination of antimicrobial therapy with compatible textiles in terms of biofunctionality is a promising innovative approach. The antibacterial effect of silver-coated textiles on S. aureus colonization has been demonstrated in an open side-to-side comparison. Silver-coated textiles were able to reduce S. aureus density significantly after 2 days of wearing, lasting until the end of treatment (day 7) and even 1 week after removal of the textiles. In addition, there was a significant difference in S. aureus density comparing silver-coated with cotton textiles. In addition, the clinical efficacy and functionality of silver-coated textiles in generalized AE have been examined in a multicenter, double-blind, placebo-controlled trial. They were able to improve objective and subjective symptoms of AE significantly within 2 weeks, showing a good wearing comfort and functionality comparable to cotton without measurable side effects. These therapeutic effects led to a significantly lower impairment of quality of life, already after 2 weeks. Beside a potent antibacterial activity in vivo, silver-coated textiles demonstrate a high efficacy in reducing the clinical severity of AE showing a wearing comfort comparable to cotton.

See <u>Thermal Suits and Wet Wraps</u> section.

Cotton: Whatever feels good on your skin, wear it. I like soft, smooth, combed cotton and silky feeling material. When it's hot, cotton is nice to absorb sweat so it doesn't burn. If you feel like a certain cotton is absorbing too much moisture, try a thinner cotton.

Satin: Satin sheets feel smooth and soft, and blood washes out easily.

Nylon: A fabric that repels moisture and oils that is hypoallergenic would be better in cooler weather. I looked for a fabric that would feel good on skin. I wanted something very smooth and slippery that wouldn't absorb the moisture or oils from my skin or make me feel itchy. I discovered that a nylon jacket (turned inside-out) was so comfortable for my skin that I didn't want to take it off. (Others felt that way when I shared the discovery with them.) Hopefully you have a smooth nylon jogging suit you can turn inside-out to see what I mean.

Why then do nylons make some feel itchy? Here's why:

"These dermatological reactions were not linked to the actual nylon fiber. Allergic Reactions to Nylon has been linked to chemicals used to inhibit bacterial growth and to azo and anthraquinone dyes used to dye the stockings brown." So, you might like to try wearing nylon next to the skin when the air is dry and where people aren't sweating from the heat.

Some Fabrics That May Aggravate Eczema

Wool can be itchy. Lanolin comes from wool. Some people wear flock lined gloves, and there can be wool in flock. If it doesn't make you feel itchy, don't worry about it.

I and others with eczema have also noticed that acrylic sweaters make us feel itchy. A chemist friend of mine says it's a very hairy fiber, and that's why it can feel itchy.

Regarding polyester, it is known for its oil-absorbing quality. There is a kitchen utensil that looks like a mop made of polyester that is used to absorb oil from the top of spaghetti sauce. However, if the fabric feels soft, smooth and silky, just where what feels good. (smiles)

Elastic and rubber can also aggravate eczema, but it just depends on what one is sensitive to.

Laundering

Some people don't use soap to wash their clothes; water is a cleanser. Some use pure baking soda. If you use laundry soap, use a brand that's "Free and Clear" or "For Sensitive Skin" and use a little less than recommended ... try running it through an extra rinse cycle. You can add 1 cup of white vinegar during the 1st rinse cycle and before the 2nd rinse cycle to help remove soap residue.

Blood Stains: Hydrogen peroxide bubbles the blood right out of clothing without discoloring fabric, but test first just for the sake of it.

See also the Dry Eczema section.

Gloves

Wearing gloves to protect yourself from water, soap and other chemicals as well as from the drying effects of things like dusting and folding clothes is important. I know so many people with terrible eczema on their hands that still immerse their hands in soapy water when washing things. Even plain water is drying on the skin.

The problem I encountered is that rubber and latex gloves and vinyl gloves irritated my skin and made them burn and itch, and cotton gloves just absorbed the moisture out of my skin. I found that the very cheap, disposable, thin, clear, plastic gloves didn't hurt my skin. I used the ones with little breathing holes in them when I did dry work so the hands wouldn't sweat too much; and, for wet work I used them under other gloves to protect the skin. I got them from my local grocery store. They use them in the bakery and the deli. I asked them if I could buy them, but they just give them to me for free.

Using cotton under latex is helpful for many. Now that I managed to get rid of the eczema on my hands (see the Bacteria section), I can use any kind of gloves without bother. I don't even use gloves sometimes anymore ...

Hand Eczema

We'd better start by saying that the good bacteria will fight the bad bacteria. So many people believe they need to wash their hands every time they touch something. Remember that preserving the good bacteria that you have on your hands will fight the bad bacteria. Also, very important is to restore the pH to the skin, and that in and of itself will help fight infections. pH balanced products are important. Now, we know that taking antibiotics all the time is not good; and, in the same way, I don't like using antibacterial soap unless there is a reason like an infection (in which case tea tree oil can be helpful, too). Water is also a cleanser, and it does dry the skin.

Preservation of the natural oils is best. When my hands are dry, I use the very thin plastic gloves with breathing holes in them (so the skin doesn't sweat so much) to protect my hands. Rubber and vinyl gloves irritated my skin, and cotton gloves absorbed the moisture out of my hands. Instead of using a lot of oil to moisturize, I used the plastic gloves for short periods of time, because it helps moisturize by cutting down on moisture loss. I use them to preserve my natural oils when folding laundry.

Check out the <u>Bacteria</u> section to see how some forms of eczema have cleared up with the use of antibacterials and antifungals.

Try not to leave gloves on all day long. The skin needs to breathe.

Cuticles

Since I quit using regular soaps, I have cuticles again. I hadn't seen my cuticles in a long time. My fingernail even grew back after it was half way gone for a couple of years, and the deep ridges smoothed over. The cuticle is the root of the fingernail; and, when eczema eats away at the cuticle, the growth of the fingernail can sometimes be impaired.

Lips

Ring Around The Lips

Toothpaste and things coming into contact with the lips can be troublesome for irritated and dry lips. I used to have a big ring around my mouth for a few years until I learned that it was the petroleum jelly that was contributing to that problem in my case. Watch for lanolin in chap sticks, too, because that can aggravate the eczema sometimes.

Lip Care

Try not to lick your lips when eating, because when food or drinks touched my lips, it burned. You can drink with a straw to avoid getting the drinks on your lips. Use a cloth to dry them when eating instead of licking them. For years, I was always putting things on my lips to make them better. Avoiding toothpaste on the lips and avoiding petroleum jelly took care of that problem.

V. INTERNAL CARE

Diet

Although nearly any food can cause an allergic reaction, a few foods account for about 90% of reactions. Among adults these foods are peanuts, nuts, fish and shellfish. Among children, they are egg, milk, peanuts, soy, and wheat.

I used to think what I ate didn't affect my skin ... then I began to study how nutrition can affect the performance of our bodies. It didn't take a genius to understand the connection between nutrition and health, and I realized that nutrition can greatly affect the largest organ of our bodies, the skin. Research shows how all different kinds of minerals, vitamins, proteins, fats, enzymes and acids can work together and affect the immune system, our skin, bacteria and sensitivities to stress.

Just as we realize that the external chemicals that come in contact with our skin affect the skin, we know that the things we consume internally will affect our skin, see: World's Healthiest Foods to research the foods you eat and how they affect health. Here's a great site that can teach you how to incorporate healthy bacteria into your diet with foods: Body Ecology Diet and another site that sells Rejuvenative Foods. Also, when you visit the Eczema Mall (under construction), check out the Food Store there and learn about the raw food diet and the "Eating for Beauty" book that's in the Food Store, and check out Supermodel's Carol Alt's Raw Food Diet article.

Considerations for People with Eczema

- Some people do better without wheat, see why in the Celiac section.

- Increase essential fatty acids like those in flaxseeds.

- Green drinks, like drinking blended kale, (see this link on kale, too) are helpful to get vitamins/minerals and to detoxify.

- Citrus tends to make some people flare up.

- Increase immune system calming foods.

- Use Grade B Maple Syrup instead of refined sugars.\

- Cut down on white breads and substitute with whole grain breads.

- Dairy products can make some people flare up, but yogurt doesn't.

- Consume more raw fruits and vegetables for enzymes, nutrients and digestion.

- Drink more water and cut down on sodas, alcohol and coffee.

- Tomatoes can make some people flare up (they are alkaline raw and acidic when cooked) .

- Salt is alkalizing and is a strong natural antihistamine.

Refined table salt is stripped of 82 of the 84 minerals salt has. Celtic salt is best and is found in health food stores. You can try No-salt (rich in potassium). Iodized salt makes some flare up.

➢ See the Bacteria section; visit the Alkaline Diet and the Enzyme sections.

See information about Food Allergy Tests, and learn what's going on with Leaky Gut Syndrome.

Considerations for Those with Candida

If you suspect candida, you may visit the Candida section for further information. Cutting down on sugars, yeasts, vinegar, dairy and increasing increase raw vegetables can be helpful.

Maple Syrup vs. White Refined Sugar

The regular use of white refined sugar can create constant imbalances which in turn will adversely affect the normal function of the liver, pancreas and spleen. These organs are important in detoxification and digestion. Special note: See how cinnamon prevents Type 2 diabetes.

Like natural fruits and vegetables, Grade B Maple Syrup is a balanced sugar and does not have the side effects that white refined sugar have. It also has a large variety of minerals and vitamins: sodium, potassium, calcium, magnesium, manganese, iron, copper, phosphorus, sulfur, chlorine and silicon, vitamin A, B1, B2, B6, C, nicotinic acid, and pantothenic acid.

A delightful snack that tastes a lot like chocolate is ground (always grind) flaxseeds mixed with the maple syrup.

Drinking Water

Here's a dehydration researcher who describes how water may cure most diseases: www.watercure.com.

I follow the above site's recommendation and do the following. As an adult, I drink 3 to 4 quarts of water a day in between meals. Further, for every quart of water, I add 1/4 teaspoon celtic salt (not regular salt) to my meals. Remember 8 oz = 1 cup; 32 oz = 4 cups = 1 quart. So, I'm drinking a 32 oz mug of water 3 to 4 x day and salting my meals. Wait 1/2 hour after drinking a quart of water before you eat, and then don't drink with your meals. Wait 2 to 2 1/2 hours after eating before drinking your next quart of water. Here's why ... and try and read the salt links above, too:

Every cell process in the body requires water. When internal water reserves are low, the body draws water away from the surface of your skin, so you need to drink a lot of water to have plump, healthy, moist skin. Water is the most important element in nourishing your body and flushes toxins out of your body. Unfortunately, the majority of people are walking around dehydrated. Drinking water will improve the condition of your skin.

What Kind of Water?

Filtered water and you can use alkaline drops purchased from the health food store if you want.

Alkalizing

Internal pH is highly important. Although externally our skin is supposed to be acidic, internally we are supposed to be alkaline. Unfortunately, in many cases it is reversed.

If you were to compare your body to a fish tank, it is easy to understand just how important a pH balanced environment is. An overly-acidic internal condition will result in an emergency expulsion of acid toxins via the skin and thus eczema. This is key: only by alkalizing your system internally will your body have the proper environment to be well. Did you know that the NIH says metabolic acidosis is common in babies fed cow-based milk formula? That's one reason so many babies have eczema.

Here's a simple article on the Alkaline Diet to start you out. See, also, the <u>Immune System Calming Foods</u> section, and you can study about alkalizing on the Internet and get a book called Sick and Tired by Dr. Robert O. Young, Ph.D. in Microbiology, Biochemistry and Nutrition.

<u>The Information Free Diet Plan</u> by Monica Reinagel is like an acid/alkaline dictionary and by far the best resource I've seen on this subject.

Alkaline and Acidic Food Chart

The anti-inflammatory diet is an alkaline diet. Shift Your pH Toward Alkaline. This chart is for those trying to "adjust" their body pH. The pH scale is from 0 to 14, with numbers below 7 acidic (low on oxygen) and numbers above 7 alkaline. An acidic body is a sickness magnet. See, also, the <u>Drink Water</u> section for information on alkalizing drops.

This chart is intended only as a general guide to alkalizing and acidifying foods.

ALKALIZING VEGETABLES
Alfalfa
Barley Grass
Beets
Beet Greens
Broccoli
Cabbage
Carrot
Cauliflower
Celery
Chard Greens
Chlorella
Collard Greens
Cucumber
Dandelions
Dulce
Edible Flowers
Eggplant
Fermented Veggies
Garlic
Green Beans
Green Peas
Kale
Kohlrabi
Lettuce
Mushrooms
Mustard Greens
Nightshade Veggies
Onions
Parsnips (high glycemic)
Peas
Peppers
Pumpkin
Radishes
Rutabaga
Sea Veggies
Spinach, green
Spirulina
Sprouts

Sweet Potatoes
Tomatoes
Watercress
Wheat Grass
Wild Greens

ALKALIZING FRUITS
Apple
Apricot
Avocado
Banana (high glycemic)
Berries
Blackberries
Cantaloupe
Cherries, sour
Coconut, fresh
Currants
Dates, dried
Figs, dried
Grapes
Grapefruit
Honeydew Melon
Lemon
Lime
Muskmelons
Nectarine
Orange
Peach
Pear
Pineapple
Raisins
Raspberries
Rhubarb
Strawberries
Tangerine
Tomato
Tropical Fruits
Umeboshi Plums
Watermelon

ALKALIZING PROTEIN
Almonds
Chestnuts

Millet
Tempeh (fermented)
Tofu (fermented)
Whey Protein Powder

ALKALIZING SWEETENERS
Stevia

ALKALIZING SPICES & SEASONINGS
Cinnamon
Curry
Ginger
Mustard
Chili Pepper
Sea Salt
Miso
Tamari
All Herbs

ALKALIZING OTHER
Apple Cider Vinegar
Bee Pollen
Lecithin Granules
Molasses, blackstrap
Probiotic Cultures
Soured Dairy Products
Green Juices
Veggie Juices
Fresh Fruit Juice
Mineral Water
Alkaline Antioxidant Water

ALKALIZING MINERALS
Cesium: pH 14
Potassium: pH 14
Sodium: pH 14
Calcium: pH 12
Magnesium: pH 9

Although it might seem that citrus fruits would have an acidifying effect on the body, the citric acid they contain actually has an alkalinizing effect in the system.

ACIDIFYING VEGETABLES
Corn
Lentils
Olives
Winter Squash

ACIDIFYING FRUITS
Blueberries
Canned or Glazed Fruits
Cranberries
Currants
Plums**
Prunes**

ACIDIFYING GRAINS, GRAIN PRODUCTS
Amaranth
Barley
Bran, wheat
Bran, oat
Corn
Cornstarch
Hemp Seed Flour
Kamut
Oats (rolled)
Oatmeal
Quinoa
Rice (all)
Rice Cakes
Rye
Spelt
Wheat
Wheat Germ
Noodles
Macaroni
Spaghetti
Bread
Crackers, soda
Flour, white
Flour, wheat

ACIDIFYING BEANS & LEGUMES
Black Beans
Chick Peas
Green Peas
Kidney Beans
Lentils
Pinto Beans
Red Beans
Soy Beans
Soy Milk
White Beans
Rice Milk
Almond Milk

ACIDIFYING DAIRY
Butter
Cheese
Cheese, Processed
Ice Cream
Ice Milk

ACIDIFYING NUTS & BUTTERS
Cashews
Legumes
Peanuts
Peanut Butter
Pecans
Tahini
Walnuts

ACIDIFYING ANIMAL PROTEIN
Bacon
Beef
Carp
Clams
Cod
Corned Beef
Fish
Haddock
Lamb
Lobster
Mussels
Organ Meats

Oyster
Pike
Pork
Rabbit
Salmon
Sardines
Sausage
Scallops
Shrimp
Scallops
Shellfish
Tuna
Turkey
Veal
Venison

ACIDIFYING FATS & OILS
Avocado Oil
Butter
Canola Oil
Corn Oil
Hemp Seed Oil
Flax Oil
Lard
Olive Oil
Safflower Oil
Sesame Oil
Sunflower Oil

ACIDIFYING SWEETENERS
Carob
Sugar
Corn Syrup

ACIDIFYING ALCOHOL
Beer
Spirits
Hard Liquor
Wine

ACIDIFYING OTHER FOODS
Catsup
Cocoa

Coffee
Vinegar
Mustard
Pepper
Soft Drinks

ACIDIFYING DRUGS & CHEMICALS
Aspirin
Chemicals
Drugs, Medicinal
Drugs, Psychedelic
Pesticides
Herbicides
Tobacco

ACIDIFYING JUNK FOOD
Coca-Cola: pH 2
Beer: pH 2.5
Coffee: pH 4

** These foods leave an alkaline ash but have an acidifying effect on the body.

UNKNOWN: There are several versions of the Acidic and Alkaline Food chart to be found in different books and on the Internet. The following foods are sometimes attributed to the Acidic side of the chart and sometimes to the Alkaline side. Remember, you don't need to adhere strictly to the Alkaline side of the chart, just make sure a good percentage of the foods you eat come from that side.

Asparagus
Brazil Nuts
Brussel Sprouts
Buckwheat
Chicken
Corn
Cottage Cheese
Eggs
Flax Seeds
Green Tea
Herbal Tea

Honey
Kombucha
Lima Beans
Maple Syrup
Milk
Nuts
Organic Milk
(unpasteurized)
Potatoes, white
Pumpkin Seeds
Sauerkraut
Soy Products
Sprouted Seeds
Squashes
Sunflower Seeds
Yogurt

Ranked Foods: Alkaline to Acidic

Here's a chart that ranks foods from most alkaline to most acidic.

Extremely Alkaline
Lemons, Watermelon

Alkaline Forming
Cantaloupe, Cayenne Celery, Dates, Figs, Kelp, Limes, Mango, Melons, Papaya, Parsley, Seaweeds, Seedless Grapes (sweet), Watercress

Asparagus, Fruit Juices, Grapes (sweet), Kiwifruit, Passion fruit, Pears (sweet), Pineapple, Raisins, Umeboshi Plums, Vegetable Juices

Moderately Alkaline
Apples (sweet), Alfalfa Sprouts, Apricots, Avocados, Bananas (ripe), Currants, Dates, Figs (fresh), Garlic, Grapefruit, Grapes (less sweet), Guavas, Herbs (leafy green), Lettuce (leafy green), Nectarine, Peaches (sweet), Pears (less sweet), Peas (fresh, sweet), Pumpkin (sweet), Sea Salt (vegetable)

Apples (sour), Beans (fresh, green), Beets, Bell Peppers, Broccoli, Cabbage, Carob, Cauliflower, Ginger (fresh), Grapes (sour), Lettuce (pale green), Oranges, Peaches (less sweet), Peas (less sweet), Potatoes (with skin), Pumpkin (less sweet), Raspberries, Strawberries, Squash, Sweet Corn (fresh), Turnip, Vinegar (apple cider)

Slightly Alkaline
Almonds, Artichokes (Jerusalem), Brussel Sprouts, Cherries, Coconut (fresh), Cucumbers, Eggplant, Honey (raw), Leeks, Mushrooms, Okra, Olives (ripe), Onions, Pickles (homemade), Radishes, Sea Salt, Spices, Tomatoes (sweet), Vinegar (sweet brown rice)

Chestnuts (dry, roasted), Egg Yolks (soft cooked), Essence Bread, Goat's Milk and Whey (raw), Mayonnaise (homemade), Olive Oil, Sesame Seeds (whole), Soy Beans (dry), Soy Cheese, Soy Milk, Sprouted Grains, Tofu, Tomatoes (less sweet), Yeast (nutritional flakes)

Neutral
Butter (fresh, unsalted), Cream (fresh, raw), Cow's Milk and Whey (raw), Margarine, Oils (except olive), Yogurt (plain)

Moderately Acidic
Bananas (green), Barley (rye), Blueberries, Bran, Butter, Cereals (unrefined), Cheeses, Crackers (unrefined rye, rice and wheat), Cranberries, Dried Beans (mung, adzuki, pinto, kidney, garbanzo), Dry Coconut, Egg Whites, Eggs Whole (cooked hard), Fructose, Goat's Milk (homogenized), Honey (pasteurized), Ketchup, Maple Syrup (unprocessed), Milk (homogenized), Molasses (unsulfured and organic), Most Nuts, Mustard, Oats (rye, organic), Olives (pickled), Pasta (whole grain), Pastry (whole grain and honey), Plums, Popcorn (with salt and/or butter), Potatoes, Prunes, Rice (basmati and brown), Seeds (pumpkin, sunflower), Soy Sauce, Wheat Bread (sprouted organic)

Extremely Acidic
Artificial Sweeteners, Beef, Beer, Breads, Brown Sugar, Carbonated Soft Drinks, Cereals (refined), Chocolate, Cigarettes and Tobacco, Coffee, Cream of Wheat (unrefined), Custard (with white sugar), Deer, Drugs, Fish, Flour (white wheat), Fruit Juices

with Sugar, Jams, Jellies, Lamb, Liquor, Maple Syrup (processed), Molasses (sulphured), Pasta (white), Pastries and Cakes from White Flour, Pickles (commercial), Pork, Poultry, Seafood, Sugar (white), Table Salt (refined and iodized), Tea (black), White Bread, White Vinegar (processed), Whole Wheat Foods, Wine, Yogurt (sweetened)

Essential Fatty Acids

Good Fats

Important: Remember that people with eczema may need to supplement with lipase enzymes to break down the fats.

Essential fatty acids ("EFAs") (also known as Vitamin F) are the fatty acids--basic building blocks of which fats and oils are composed--that the body cannot make. EFAs are required for maintaining the structure of cell membranes and the permeability of the skin. Some of the major functions of EFAs are:

- insulation for your body against heat loss

- prevention of your skin from drying or flaking

- a cushion for your tissues and organs

- production of "prostaglandin" families, hormones necessary for cell to cell biochemical functions

There are two EFAs in the human diet: alpha-linolenic acid (the parent fatty acid of the Omega-3 family) and linoleic acid (the parent fatty acid of the Omega-6 family). Omega-6 is the class of EFAs found most commonly in the American diet, but Omega-3 is sorely lacking in many diets.

Fat Facts

Part of the reason fats and oils have earned such a bad reputation in recent years is because people eat too much fat; however, many people don't realize that in North America most people consume only 20% of EFAs required for optimal health. In fact, EFAs are considered valuable in weight management and weight loss. Specialized fat cells, which comprise roughly 10% of total body fat, are capable of burning approximately 1/4 of calories consumed. It takes fat to lose fat.

EFAs are the only fats that become prostaglandins, which play a key role in regulating the immune system.

Eczema and EFAs

The National Institute of Health ("NIH") sent me a draft of their Handout on Atopic Dermatitis for my comments. It states,

> *"Biochemical Abnormalities: Scientists suspect that changes in the skin's protective barrier make people with atopic dermatitis more sensitive to irritants. Such people have lower levels of fatty acids (substances that provide moisture and elasticity) in their skin, which causes dryness and reduces the skin's ability to control inflammation .... Scientists are focusing on identifying new treatments for atopic dermatitis including ... fatty acid supplements ...."*

It further states ...

> *"In people with atopic dermatitis, monocytes appear to play a role in the decreased production of an immune system hormone called interferon gamma ("IFN-y"), which helps regulate allergic reactions. This defect may cause exaggerated immune and inflammatory responses in the blood and tissues of people with atopic dermatitis."*

92

"Researchers also think that an imbalance in the immune system may contribute to the development of atopic dermatitis. It appears that the part of the immune system responsible for stimulating IgE is overactive, and the part that makes IFN-γ and handles skin viral and fungal infections is not working sufficiently. Indeed, the skin of people with atopic dermatitis shows increased susceptibility to skin infections. This imbalance appears to result in the skin's inability to restrain dermatitis, or inflammation, even in areas of skin that appear normal."

NIH's final copy of their handbook on atopic dermatitis is out, and you can see it here.

Technically Speaking

Flaxseed favorably influences immune response. The flaxseed component alpha-linolenic acid ("ALA") alters membrane phospholipids, inhibits arachidonic acid biosynthesis from linoleic acid, inhibits the production of proinflammatory eicosanoids from arachidonic acid, and suppresses lymphocyte proliferation and cytokine production. Flaxseed lignans are potent inhibitors of platelet-activating factor, a mediator of inflammation. Through these effects, flaxseed has the potential to be used for the treatment of disorders characterized in part by activated lymphocytes and a hyper-stimulated immune response. Such disorders include rheumatoid arthritis, eczema, psoriasis, multiple sclerosis and systemic lupus erythematosus.

Omega-3 fatty acids modify immune and inflammatory reactions. The key to a healthy immune system is found in EFAs. EFAs common to flaxseed oil are ultimately converted to hormone-like substances known as prostaglandins, and are important for the regulation of a host of bodily functions including:

- inflammation, pain and swelling
- secretions from mucus membranes and their viscosity
- water retention
- blood clotting ability
- allergic response and rheumatoid arthritis
- nerve transmission
- steroid production and hormone synthesis

See, the Flaxseed section. Great Smokies Diagnostic Lab has an Essential and Metabolic Fatty Acids Analysis section.

Three Notes

1. To help you get the most out of flaxseed oil, try to limit the refined oils you consume. This includes hydrogenated oils. These oils are metabolized in the same pathways as the natural oils and can block their functions. Moderation is good, nothing radical.

2. There are special proteins in yogurt or cottage cheese (non-fat or low-fat) that enhance the properties of the EFA's; so, mixing the oil with either one is beneficial.

3. Vitamins A, C, E, B-2, B-3, B-6, Pantothenic acid, B-12, biotin, and minerals calcium, magnesium, potassium, sulfur, and zinc are all involved in EFA metabolism. Zinc seems necessary for at least two stages in EFA metabolism, the conversion of linoleic acid to gamma-linolenic acid, and the mobilization of dihomogammalinolenic acid (DGLA) for the synthesis of 1 series PGs.

Taking a good multivitamin and mineral supplement with special attention to B-6 is recommended.

Flax Oil and Flaxseed

Important: Remember that people with atopic eczema have trouble metabolizing fats and will benefit from supplementing with enzymes to break down the fats.

How I Discovered Flax Oil Helps Eczema

I did an electronic search in the Bible for the word "skin" to see what I could find to help us with eczema. Verses about linen and flax came up as a result of that search (linen comes from flaxseed). So, I started looking into flax and linen to see how they could help eczema. What I found was miraculous!

Linen is the oldest textile material in the world. Its history goes back many thousands of years, well into the Stone Age. Flax has been eaten by the human race for over 5,000 years. In 5,000 BC flax was cultivated in Babylon. In the 11th Century, it was used to help cure many skin diseases, including leprosy.

The miracle is that flax is the richest source of Omega 3 essential fatty acids at 57% (over two times the amount of Omega-3 fatty acids as fish oils). Flax oil requires less processing and costs 80% less than fish oil. Unrefined organic flax oil is also a rich source of electrons.

Benefits

Flaxseed is also one of the richest sources of lignans, a type of phytoestrogen which may protect against cancer, particularly hormone-sensitive cancers such as those of the breast and prostate.

Flaxseed contains essential vitamins and minerals. It is particularly rich in potassium, providing about seven times as much as a banana on a dry-weight basis.

From Prescription for Nutritional Healing by Dr. James Balch and Phyllis Balch, CNC, flaxseed:

> *Flaxseed promotes strong bones, nails, and teeth, as well as healthy skin. Used for colon problems, female disorders and inflammation. Flaxseeds are rich in omega-3 essential fatty acids, magnesium, potassium, and fiber. They are also a good source of the B vitamins, protein, and zinc. They are low in saturated fats and calories, and contain no cholesterol; and, as a matter of fact, flax oil decreases probability of heart attack and stroke, because it helps keep the arteries clean and free of plaque and cholesterol.*

EFAs are necessary/crucial for infants, nursing mothers, and children.

How Soon Will It Make A Difference?

The following were typical periods of time in which subjects of a pilot study noted the beneficial effects of the Omega-3 flaxseed supplements. A long wait is not always necessary before the results are visible:

Time after taking oil supplement:

<u>2 Hours</u>: Mood improved, feeling of calm, depression relieved.

<u>2-7 Days</u>: Skin smoother, with less flaking and scaling; backs of hands and fingers smoother.

<u>2-14 Days</u>: Relief for disturbed mental patients; relief from feelings of anxiety.

<u>2-6 Weeks</u>: Osteoarthritis relieved, with easier movements and less inflammation and pain. Bursitis and other soft

tissue inflammations reduced. Tinnitus and noises in the ears subside. Dandruff and flaking of the scalp less noticeable; dry skin alleviated.

2-4 Months: Rheumatoid pain diminished. "Easy bruising" reduced. Choking spasms subside. Fewer muscular spasms; no nighttime leg cramps; relief from ocular spasms. Relief from itching and burning sensations. Improved skin color. Reduced sun sensitivity.

3-6 Months: Diminished food allergies. Healing of chronic infections. Disappearance of rough, bumpy skin on upper arms. Improved alcohol tolerance. Improved cold tolerance. Lessening of fatigue. Increased calm and feeling of well-being."

How Much Flax Oil We Should Take?

Some people prefer to take capsules as opposed to oil. Whatever your preference, please be aware of the following:

Oil: One tablespoon of flax oil per 100 lbs. is recommended. There are 14 grams of flax oil in one tablespoon. If you weigh closer to 200 pounds, 2 tablespoons per day is recommended. Since 3 teaspoons = 1 tablespoon, 1 1/2 teaspoons would be recommended for children who weigh 50 lbs.

I dip my tortillas in flax oil (salted) ... and I love it. Hard for me to take it any other way.

Capsules: Since, flax capsules come in 1,000 mg, between ten and fourteen capsules per day for adults is recommended. 1,000 mg = 1 gram.

Three Final Notes

1. To help you get the most out of flaxseed oil, try to limit the refined oils you consume. This includes hydrogenated oils. These oils are metabolized in the same pathways as the natural oils and can block their functions. Moderation is good.

2. There are special proteins in yogurt or cottage cheese (non-fat or low-fat) that enhance the properties of the EFA's; so, mixing the oil with either one is beneficial.

3. Vitamins A, C, E, B-2, B-3, B-6, Pantothenic acid, B-12, biotin, and minerals calcium, magnesium, potassium, sulfur, and zinc are all involved in EFA metabolism. Taking a good multivitamin and mineral supplement with special attention to B-6 is recommended.

Hydrochloric Acid Deficiency

In chronic eczema the severity of the condition seems to correlate with the extent of stomach hydrochloric acid ("HCl") deficiency, and decreased HCl is also associated with vitamin B group deficiency. General allergies, and specifically food allergies, are correlated with low HCl. Poor food breakdown and the "leaky gut" syndrome are associated with food allergies.

Hydrochloric Acid is a digestive acid secreted by a healthy stomach when food is eaten. It initiates the digestion of proteins, fats, and carbohydrates and aids in the absorption of several vitamins and minerals. In addition, because HCl is a strong acid, it inhibits the growth of harmful bacteria. HCl kills various bacteria from food which may pose a health hazard, inactivates the salivary amylase from the mouth, and activates pepsin, an enzyme which starts protein digestion in the stomach. HCl also denatures protein, or chemically alters the structure of protein to make protein more digestible. Acids, chemicals, heat, and radiation are various ways proteins are denatured.

When someone has a HCl Deficiency, their body is deficient in mineral salts that are used to produce HCl. You see, the good news is that a mineral like potassium not only stimulates the production of hydrochloric acid (which favors digestion) but it also contributes to a balanced pH level in the blood.

The most carefully planned diet fails to accomplish its purpose unless digestion and absorption are adequate and normal. Digestive enzymes and HCl must be produced in adequate amounts to facilitate normal digestion. Too little HCl inhibits protein digestion and the absorption of vitamin C causes the destruction of vitamin B-complex factors and prevents essential calcium, iron and other minerals from being assimilated to the extent that anemia and bone fragility may develop. A large variety of nutritional deficiencies may restrict the production of essential enzymes allowing putrefactive bacteria to multiply in tremendous amounts forming great quantities of stomach and intestinal gas. Further, a deficiency or absence of normal beneficial bacteria in the intestinal tract will allow propagation of gas-forming and disease and odor-forming bacteria.

Low stomach acid may be the result of heredity, extended use of drugs such as antacids, anti-ulcer medications (cimetidine, ranitidine and others), infection in the gut, or food allergies (especially to milk and dairy products). Drinking milk with meals stops the production of HCL. Having lemon with your meal is helpful. Doctors specializing in nutritional medicine can do several tests to determine the etiology. One of these is the comprehensive digestive and stool analysis ("CDSA").

Magnesium, Hydrochloric Acid and Digestion

Magnesium is needed to reduce histamine levels. In the book Encyclopedia of Natural Medicine, the authors note that food allergies are usually associated with low hydrochloric acid levels and poor digestion. The authors' rationale for this is that low stomach acid leaves food undigested and fermenting in the intestinal tract. This fermentation causes gas, bloating and stomach upset, the symptoms of irritable bowel syndrome. Undigested and fermented food causes the body to raise histamine levels, which produce allergic reactions. This is why people take antihistamines for allergies, to lower histamine levels.

Low stomach acid levels reduce levels of beneficial intestinal bacteria which is needed for absorption of magnesium. When lab rats are deprived of magnesium, a wide variety of studies have noted that they develop allergy like symptoms. Their ears turn red and they develop skin problems. Rats with magnesium deficiencies have increases in histamine levels. They also have raised levels of white blood cell counts. Mg deficiency has been implicated in allergies and allergic skin reaction in many studies on humans, too. Variations of allergies, skin allergies, and raised white blood cells have been noted in many chronic disorders.

Stress stops the production of HCL. See, Magnesium.

One method used to find out if you have a stomach acid insufficiency is to look at your fingernails or toe nails and see if there are vertical ridges or lines. If the lines are strong, then there is not only a stomach acid lack but also the body is too acidic with respect to the acid/alkaline balance.

Proper Food Combining Helps Digestion

As the food enters the stomach, proteins are broken down by HCl. If you drink before, during or after a meal, the HCl in your stomach is diluted and will inhibit or slow down digestion.

Raw vegetables and fruits contain enzymes which helps to take the strain off our finite (limited) enzyme production ability.

Protein should be eaten first so that the HCl can work on them immediately. You can then eat vegetables, but do not eat any fruit (at that time). Fruits cause an alkaline substance to be excreted which inhibits protein and starch digestion.

The diet should consist of adequate amounts of fresh, raw green vegetables with some care to cut down on white refined sugar, hydrogenated fats and oils, and processed, chemicalized foods, although olive oil activates the secretion of bile and pancreatic hormones. Replacement of normal healthy-producing bacteria is a must and is accomplished by regular use of fermented foods as yogurt, raw natural sauerkraut, acidophilus milk products and probiotics.

If the cause of low stomach acid is heredity, a variety of things can be tried. These include supplements of lemon juice (and believe it or not lemons are alkalizing), vitamin B5 and vitamin B6.

Supplements

There are digestive enzymes with HCL you can buy from the health food store, and there are many herbs that aid digestion. Sulfur also stimulates bile secretion and safflowers simulate HCL production.

Zinc also assists in the production of HCL.

Leaky Gut Syndrome

"The open door you don't want. Healthy Times Spring/Summer '05

A serious strike against your health, leaky gut opens the door to a barrage of physical complaints. Here is the lowdown on this grim predicament as well as the encouraging probiotic solution.

Friendly bacteria protect the mucous lining of the intestines, forming a barrier that serves as your natural immune defense system. Conversely, harmful bacteria exude toxins that cause gut inflammation and weaken the normally tight junctions of the gut wall cells. Toxins, unfriendly bacteria, food proteins, yeasts and abnormal immune stimulating chemicals can then permeate the compromised gut barrier. This is Leaky Gut Syndrome - a serious affront to your health.

In an ironic twist, antibiotic therapy contributes to this dilemma by killing both detrimental and protective bacteria, leaving an open playing field for a proliferation of harmful microorganisms to mount their attack.

Bacteria and yeast invade the bloodstream and can initiate infection anywhere in the body. Large food proteins pass through the gut wall and the body's defense system interprets them as harmful invaders. Plaguing food allergies develop. Leakage of toxins burdens the liver, and chemical sensitivity may arise.

To counter this process, you must "plug" the leaks in your defense. How? You boost your levels of beneficial bacteria by taking probiotic supplements. When ample "friendly bacteria" are covering the intestinal walls, the invaders are not able to enter the body by penetrating the lining of the GI tract.

To slam the door on leaky gut and get back on track, you must normalize your GI microflora. L. acidophilus, NAS adhesion super strain clings to the upper intestinal walls; Bifidobacterium bifidum protects the lower intestines; and L. bulgaricus aids digestion throughout the GI system.

Effectiveness of Different Kinds of Good Bacteria

Now, in terms of the strength and livelihood of good bacteria, unrefrigerated probiotics may not be as effective as those that are refrigerated.

Enzymes

We've all heard about amino acids ... the building blocks of the body. It's great to have them, but we also need the construction workers to move those building blocks to get the work done. Consider enzymes as construction workers of the living system.

Enzymes are protein molecules that help out a chemical reaction by making it quicker and easier for the reaction to occur. They are the primary motivators of all the biochemical processes in the body. Enzymes are responsible for certain functions such as food digestion, building bones and tissues and aiding in detoxification. They digest our food and convert it so that our muscles, nerves and glands are fortified and assist kidneys, lungs, liver, skin and colon in their important eliminative tasks. They have been referred to as "very strong anti-inflammatories." Although most chemical reactions in our bodies would happen without enzymes, they would just happen very slowly.

Many people compare enzymes to locks and keys. The enzymes in your body will only work on one type of substrate. This means that if you are missing a certain kind of enzyme in your body, you may not be able to perform certain types of reactions. For instance, if someone are missing the enzyme that breaks down lactose in milk into its monosaccharide form, they can't digest milk.

With over 1000 types of enzymes, there are three broad classifications: 1) metabolic enzymes are produced in every cell of the body and perform specific biochemical reactions in the tissues and organs of the body; 2) digestive enzymes are produced by the body and are specifically used to break down or digest ingested food, and 3) food enzymes, not produced by the body, are found in raw food and liberated during digestion. The enzymes most often found in supplements are: 1) lipase to digest fats and oils, 2) protease to digest proteins, 3) amylase to digest carbohydrates, and 4) lactase to digest milk sugar or lactose.

Are You Getting Your Enzymes?

Bananas, avocados, papayas, mangos, and pineapples are examples of fruits that are high in enzymes. One of the best sources of enzymes is sprouts. Unfortunately, when food is cooked--whether it be baked, boiled, broiled, microwaved, steamed, etc.--these enzymes are destroyed. When we eat raw fruits or vegetables, each piece already contains enough enzymes to aid in its own digestion. Cooked food takes from our body's storehouse of enzymes. When we eat cooked food, enzymes that can be used for healing our bodies or maintaining our immune system are diverted and sent into the digestive system to digest our food. This is because the body puts a higher priority on digestion than on maintaining health. If we don't replenish our supply of enzymes, we can become enzyme deficient.

Digestion and Eczema

The Physician's Handbook of Clinical Nutritional states that improving digestion is essential in patients with eczema. In The Hydrochloric Acid section we learned that digestive enzymes and HCL must be produced in adequate amounts to facilitate normal digestion. We also learned that good bacteria are key in aiding digestion, and nutritional deficiencies may restrict the production of essential enzymes.

I've noticed for years that sometimes I looked pregnant when I wasn't. Then, the bloating would just go away, and I couldn't figure it out at first. I learned that irritable bowel syndrome ("IBS") is one of the most common disorders of the digestive tract, and symptoms include abdominal bloating, pain, gas and irregular bowel habits. For years I had to avoid foods like beans and ice cream, because they made my stomach uncomfortable. Now, though, with enzymes I don't have those symptoms anymore.

Supplementing With Enzymes

When I began eating more raw vegetables like broccoli, it did bother my stomach. Foods like beans, whole grain cereals, broccoli, cabbage, cauliflower, brussel sprouts, onions, lentils, green peppers, cucumbers and many other healthful foods contain certain complex sugars "which we cannot digest". The undigested sugars ferment inside the body causing gassiness.

Another very helpful enzyme is the lactase enzyme. If your stomach gets uncomfortable when eating things like cottage cheese and ice cream, you might lack lactase enzymes. Lactase enzymes give your body extra help to break down the milk sugar found in many dairy foods and makes dairy foods more digestible.

Enzymes are not drugs, they don't have bad side effects, the body will eliminate whatever it doesn't need, they are safe, don't interfere with any medication and are non-toxic.

Did you know that panic disorder and multiple chemical sensitivity may be attributed to enzyme deficiencies?

Supplements - The Nutritional Orchestra

The Physicians Handbook of Clinical Nutrition ("PHCN") lists various supplements for eczema. I noticed that nutrition helped control the eczema. You may like to visit the <u>Diet</u> section to see what I'm doing. My skin is better. After researching how nutrition affects the skin, it's no wonder.

I want to make this easy, because it is. I used to get lost in it all, but then it all pieced together like an orchestra of nutrients. Here it is in a nutshell: whole food sources are the best, and just remember what granny always used to say, "Be sure and eat your green leafy vegetables!"

For Supplements, Refer to the Following Sections:
B-Vitamins
Bacteria
Detoxifiers
Diet
Drinking Water
Enzymes
Essential Fatty Acids
Herbs
Hydrochloric Acid
Magnesium

Vitamins and Minerals

Vitamin A

Vitamin A is essential to maintain intact epithelial tissues as a physical barrier to infection. It is essential for the correct functioning, development and maintenance of epithelial cells. These cells form the outer layer of the skin. Promotes tissue healing, strengthens and protects the skin tissue and fights infection which is implicated in eczema. When applied topically, it is found to rapidly improve the epithelial barrier function from damage caused by chemical irritation or inflammation.

Vitamin A and its derivatives (retinol, retinoic acid, retinaldehyde) have an anti-ageing effect when applied to the skin. They accelerate cell renewal and stimulate the production of keratinocytes and fibroblasts as well as collagen. Retinoids suppress impaired elastic fibres and thus encourage a reduction in wrinkles and fine lines as well as improvement in the skin's biomechanical properties. They increase dermal vascularisation, and by renewing keratinocytes, reduce pigmented spots. The skin looks more delicate, with a better color, less wrinkled, in short – it looks younger and more attractive.

The Vitamin A oil I used at first was Spring Valley, Vitamin A, 8000 I.U. made with soybean and fish oil--Soybean oil is not allergenic to soybean-sensitive individuals. I just cut open the capsules and put it on my hands. At first, it seemed like my skin improved. Within a day or so, though, I broke out with a rash (maybe from the soybean), and the same thing happened to my neighbor (who suffers from eczema). Later researched showed that topical soybean oil actually delays repair of the barrier function along with olive oil, but sunflower oil helped repair it.

I'm researching and testing on myself and others African Red Palm Oil. Red palm oil is red due to the high content of beta carotene (15 times higher than carrots). Since the color can stain, wear darker clothes. If you're putting it on your hands, wear the food service handles gloves. Find it in your health foods stores like Wild Oats. Topical beta-carotene penetrated well into human epidermis and induced a 10-fold increase of epidermal retinyl esters, which demonstrates that topical beta-carotene is converted into retinyl esters by human epidermis and thus appears as a precursor of epidermal vitamin A. See NIH report. It helps prevent asthma attacks. Vitamin A is also found in alfalfa, borage leaves, burdock root, cayenne, chickweed, hops, nettle, parsley, peppermint, raspberry leaf, red clover, rose hips and yellow dock.

B Vitamins

The B-complex is a collective group of water-soluble vitamins. They are called a "complex" because they need each other, work together, complement each other and are often found together in foods.

Below are some benefits derived from taking B vitamins for eczema. Herbs where they can be found are also listed.

Vitamin B-1 (Thiamine)

Helps maintain a healthy nervous system. Assists in production of hydrochloric acid. Found in alfalfa, burdock root, catnip, cayenne, chamomile, chickweed, fenugreek, hops, nettle, parsley, peppermint, raspberry leaf, red clover, rose hips and yellow dock

Vitamin B-2 (Riboflavin)

Promotes healthy skin, hair and nails. Aids in the metabolism of fats. Eliminates dandruff. Facilitates use of oxygen in skin tissue. Found in alfalfa, burdock, catnip, cayenne, chamomile, chickweed, fenugreek, hops, nettle, parsley, peppermint, raspberry leaves, red clover, rose hips and yellow dock.

Vitamin B-3 (Niacin/Niacinamide/Nicotinic Acid)

Needed for proper circulation, healthy skin. Aids in proper function of the nervous and digestive systems. Assists in the production of hydrochloric acid. Found in alfalfa, burdock root, catnip, cayenne, chamomile, chickweed, hops, licorice, nettle, parsley, peppermint, raspberry leaf, red clover, rosehips, slippery elm and yellow dock

Vitamin B-5 (Pantothenic Acid)

Known as "the anti-stress vitamin." Vital for proper functioning of the adrenal glands and formation of antibodies; helps convert fats, carbohydrates and protein into energy; provides a defense against stress and relief from allergies; alleviates symptoms of stiffness from arthritis and improves ability to heal and withstand physical injury.

Vitamin B-6 (Pyridoxine)

Necessary in the production of hydrochloric acid. Helps digest proteins, carbohydrates and fats; assists in the absorption of vitamin B-12, aids in maintaining potassium balance. Helpful in the treatment of allergies and arthritis. Found in alfalfa and catnip.

Vitamin B -12 (Cyancobalamin)

Assists in the growth and repair of tissue, helps maintain a healthy nervous system as well as digestive system. Prevents nerve damage. Maintains the fatty sheaths that cover and protect nerve endings. Found in alfalfa and hops.

Inositol

Helps form lecithin, metabolizes fat, helps in preventing eczema, promotes healthy hair, produces a calming effect and nourishes brain cells.

Biotin (Vitamin H)

Important coenzyme that is involved in the metabolism fats; aids cell growth; promotes healthy sweat glands and nerve tissue. It helped stop my hair from falling out and prevents candida yeast from rooting into the intestinal tract).

Vitamin C

Required for tissue growth and repair. Aids in production of anti-stress hormones. Essential in formation of collagen, a principal protein that gives the skin its structural integrity. Found in alfalfa, burdock root, cayenne, chickweed, fenugreek, hops, peppermint, nettle, parsley, raspberry leaf, red clover, rosehips, skullcap, yellow dock

Calcium

We've all learned that dairy can aggravate eczema, so we all pretty much just avoided it. We'll after my skin was great for a long time, I decided to experiment with myself and just start drinking a ton of milk. I wanted to see how badly it would break me out. I thought for sure I would get a good case of patchy eczema; but, instead, my skin got so much smoother, more hydrated, a better color that I couldn't believe it. It was the only thing I changed in my diet, and my skin took a big leap forward in improvement. Figure that one.

It was the calcium ... welcome to the wide world of calcium and how it helps skin so much so that the Winter Dry Skin isn't even a problem for me.

Read these links:

- Bion Research
- Drink Milk to Glo and for Winter Woes
- More on Calcium and Milk from Harvard

From American Chronicle: Calcium is a regulator of every organ in the body. The skin guards its calcium level very carefully and the calcium integrity of the upper epidermis regulates at least four major skin functions. Calcium regulates the lipid barrier process. High calcium content in the upper epidermis helps maintain continual and efficient barrier functions. Calcium can significantly reduce dryness.

I do drink milk now, and my skin likes it a lot. Just need to keep pH balance in check with the Acid/Alkaline Diet.

Milk Allergy Letter

Hello Christina,

I did a phone consultation with you back in the summer. I had tried many things from your book and nothing was working. I had taken my 7 year old daughter to the children's doctor several times and also to a dermatologist. Nothing they tried worked either. In late august I finally found a naturopathic doctor and took her there. She told us our daughter had a milk allergy. So, we eliminated milk from her diet and she is now 90% clear of her eczema. She has not had any new spots break out at all. She just has two small areas where the skin is still healing and will itch at times. She has improved so much, I just can't believe milk had caused her all those problems. What makes me just furious is that none of the regular doctors never cared enough to help her. She was so bad she had all of her skin just torn up from the itching. Her sheets would have blood on them in the mornings from the scratching all night long. I don't know how the doctors could just ignore something like that.

Anyways, I just wanted to say thanks for your great website, which led me to going to a naturopathic doctor. My daughter is well on her way to recovery.

Thanks and have a great day!
Patty

Vitamin E

Helps protect essential fatty acids. Necessary for tissue repair. Promotes healthy skin. Found in alfalfa, dandelion, flaxseed, nettle, raspberry leaf and rose hips

Lecithin

Needed for better absorption of the essential fatty acids. It is a component of all living cells and an integral part of all organs and glands. The brain itself contains 25% phospholipids on a dry weight basis. Phospholipids are also among the primary building blocks of all cellular membranes. Membrane functions include cellular transport of nutrients and wastes, internal cellular pressure regulation, and ion exchange.

Magnesium

Due to the association of magnesium ("Mg") with asthma, I began to research to see how it may relate to eczema. Magnesium is a metallic element which in ribbon or powder form burns with a brilliant white light. As I studied Mg,1 I found that much of my eczema research was tied by magnesium. It is an essential cofactor in more than 300 different enzymatic reactions, including carbohydrate utilization, ATP metabolism, muscle contraction, transmembrane ion transport (calcium, sodium, chloride, potassium), and the synthesis of fat, protein, and nucleic acids.

Magnesium is needed to reduce histamine levels. In the book Encyclopedia of Natural Medicine, the authors note that food allergies are usually associated with low hydrochloric acid levels and poor digestion. The authors' rationale for this is that low stomach acid leaves food undigested and fermenting in the intestinal tract. This fermentation causes gas, bloating and stomach upset, the symptoms of irritable bowel syndrome. Undigested and fermented food causes the body to raise histamine levels, which produce allergic reactions. This is why people take antihistamines for allergies, to lower histamine levels.

Low stomach acid levels reduce levels of beneficial intestinal bacteria which is needed for absorption of magnesium. When lab rats are deprived of magnesium, a wide variety of studies have noted that they develop allergy like symptoms. Their ears turn red and they develop skin problems. Rats with magnesium deficiencies have increases in histamine levels. They also have raised levels of white blood cell counts. Mg deficiency has been implicated in allergies and allergic skin reaction in many studies on humans, too. Variations of allergies, skin allergies, and raised white blood cells have all been noted as features of many chronic disorders.

What Magnesium Affects

1. Magnesium (Mg) deficiency increases sensitivity to stress, while stress aggravates magnesium deficiency. Conversely magnesium deficit creates a hyper susceptibility to stress, even in cases of chronic marginal deficit. Thus, magnesium deficit and stress reinforce each other in a pathogenic vicious circle.

2. Peptic ulcers in rats are characteristic of the early stress reaction, which sensitizes the mucosa to irritants and other stimuli, especially in Mg deficiency.

3. Allergy or pseudo allergy represent by far the most frequent expressions of marginal magnesium deficiency.

4. Mg deficiency intensifies stress ulcers through its

stimulation of histamine secretion. Mg deficiency in rats increases degranulation of mast cells with histamine release.

5.　Bronchial asthma has long been associated with hypomagnesaemia. It evokes adrenergic and cortisol, which lower Mg levels and is characterized by histamine release.

6.　Mg deficiency affects lipid metabolism and is associated with tissue injury, affecting the physical state of membrane bilayer lipids. Defective membrane function could be the primary lesion underlying cellular disturbances in Mg-deficient animals.

7.　Mg has profound effects of solute and water transport in various cells. Mg appears to be an essential factor in the regulation of the transport of potassium through the cell membranes.

8.　Mg plays an essential role in protein synthesis and is a key cofactor for hundreds of enzymes; It plays many roles at the mitochondrial level, activating numerous enzymes.

9.　Low magnesium reduces T-4 helper cells.

Magnesium's Relationships with Eczema

Stress, allergy and pseudo allergy (hives from stress), lipids (fats), potassium, the production of enzymes, corticosteroid secretion, histamine, and sensitization are all mentioned above. As we know, they all have a lot to do with eczema. Magnesium was the first thing I encountered that pulled together all of the above. So, we see that Mg deficiency can have a wide ripple effect. Alkalinity of the body, the breakdown of foods, absorption of vitamins and minerals, elimination of toxins, synthesis of fats, hormone balance, and the immune system can all be affected by magnesium.

Magnesium and Potassium

Mg loss interferes with potassium repletion. Mg has profound effects of solute and water transport in various cells and appears to be an essential factor in the regulation of the transport of potassium through the cell membranes. In the Potassium section we learned that potassium is an essential mineral that is important for controlling your body's fluid balance. It assists in the regulation of the acid-base and water balance in the blood and the body tissues and helps preserve proper alkalinity of the body's fluid. It also works with sodium to regulate the body's waste balance and normalize heart rhythms, aids in clear thinking by sending oxygen to the brain, stimulates the kidneys to eliminate poisonous body wastes, assists in reducing high blood pressure and promotes healthy skin. Initial symptoms of potassium deficiency include dry skin.

Magnesium, Stress and Hydrochloric Acid

In the Anti-Stress section we learned that stress aggravates eczema. Here we see that Mg deficiency increases sensitivity to stress. Stress stops the production of hydrochloric acid. We learned in the Hydrochloric Acid section that if hydrochloric acid is low or absent, amino acids, vitamins and minerals are poorly absorbed. The best recognized nutrient deficiency caused by low or deficient stomach acid is vitamin B12 deficiency. (B12 assists in the growth and repair of tissue, helps maintain a healthy nervous system as well as digestive system for the proper absorption of foods, protein synthesis, metabolism of fats and carbohydrates. The Physician's Handbook of Clinical Nutrition says "lack of stomach hydrochloric acid is prevalent in atopic dermatitis," and recommends enzyme supplementation.

Magnesium and Cortisol

Elevated levels of cortisol have been reported in many diseases including eczema and psoriasis. Stress intensifies release of the corticosteroid hormone. Excess corticosteroids cause Mg loss in tissue, and Mg deficiency intensifies reactions to stress.

Magnesium and Histamine

Mg deficiency in rats increases degranulation of mast cells with histamine release. In man the highest concentrations of histamine are in the skin, lungs, and GI mucosa. Histamine is present mainly in the intracellular granules of mast cells, but there is also an important extra-mast-cell pool in the gastric mucosa, with smaller amounts in the brain, heart, and other organs. When histamine is released into the bloodstream, the blood vessels swell and leak fluid into the skin and underlying tissues. This can cause the characteristic red blotches and intense itchiness.

Magnesium, Allergies, Asthma and Eczema

Eczema has been categorized with allergies and asthma. Sensitization and increased histamine production are associated with Mg deficiency. Magnesium has several anti-asthmatic actions: as a calcium antagonist it relaxes airway smooth muscle (in vitro) and dilates bronchioles (in vivo). It also inhibits cholinergic transmission, increases nitric oxide release, and reduces airway inflammation (by stabilizing mast cells and T-lymphocytes). The investigators concluded, "Low magnesium intake may therefore be involved in the etiology of asthma and chronic obstructive airways disease. Increased magnesium reduces lung hyper-reactivity.

Magnesium and Lipid Metabolism

Mg deficiency affects lipid metabolism and is associated with tissue injury, affecting the physical state of membrane bi-layers. Defective membrane function could be the primary lesion underlying cellular disturbances in Mg-deficient animals. We learned in the Flax Oil section that scientists suspect that changes in the skin's protective barrier make people with eczema more sensitive to irritants. Such people have lower levels of fatty acids (substances that provide moisture and elasticity) in their skin, which causes dryness and reduces the skin's ability to control inflammation. It was also shown that Omega-3 fatty acids modify immune and inflammatory reactions.

Daily Requirements of Magnesium

Large scale dietary surveys have disclosed that the dietary Mg intake of most Americans falls short of the daily requirement. The RDI for Mg is 400 mg daily. It must be brought to our attention that fat, sugar, salt, vitamin D, fiber, proteins, ethyl alcohol and calcium all increase the dietary requirement of Mg. In humans, sugar loading causes magnesiuresis, possibly converting a marginal intake to a deficient one. You'll know you're getting enough if your stools are soft ... too much if you get diarrhea so you just back off a little.

When to Take Magnesium

It is energizing and can have a negative impact on getting to sleep and staying asleep when taken too late. If taken early enough in the day, it often corrects insomnia.

Potassium

Potassium is an essential mineral that is important for controlling the body's fluid balance. It assists in the regulation of the acid-base and water balance in the blood and the body tissues and helps preserve proper alkalinity of the body's fluid. Initial symptoms of potassium deficiency include slow reflexes, muscle weakness, and dry skin.

Potassium is one of the most important elements in our diets. It works with sodium to regulate the body's waste balance and normalize heart rhythms, aids in clear thinking by sending oxygen to the brain, preserves proper alkalinity of body fluids, stimulates the kidneys to eliminate poisonous body wastes, assists in reducing high blood pressure and promotes healthy skin.

There is no USRDI for potassium ... health officials are currently discussing this issue. However, on food labels the RDI for potassium is listed at 3,500 mg daily. Please note that 18,000 mg daily can be toxic.

Sources of Potassium

There are products that are salt alternatives (found in the grocery store near the salt) that are made from potassium salt. (No sodium). One is called Nu-Salt and another No Salt. No salt has

650 mg or 19% of the RDI in 1/4 teaspoon and Nu-Salt has 530 mg in 1/6th teaspoon. Potassium chloride and potassium bitartrate (cream of tartar) are among the ingredients.

Doctors can prescribe potassium supplements that come in about 600 mg (but the Pharmacist says it's as big as a horse pill and coated with wax). Pharmacist agreed majority of people are way deficient in potassium and highly recommended the Nu-Salt/No-Salt route.

- A medium banana supplies 630 milligrams of potassium or about 75 milligrams per inch.
- An 8 oz glass of freshly squeezed orange juice supplies 480 milligrams of potassium.
- 1/4 cup of raisins supplies 310 milligrams of potassium.
- potato (1 medium, baked with skin) 844 mg
- kidney beans (1 cup) 713 mg
- cantaloupe (1 cup) 494 mg
- green beans (1/2 cup cooked) 185 mg
- milk (8 ounces skim) 406 mg
- yogurt (8 ounces low fat vanilla) 498 mg
- spinach (1/2 cup cooked) 419 mg
- carrots (1 medium raw) 233 mg
- watermelon (1 cup) 186 mg
- chicken breast (3 oz without skin, cooked) 220 mg
- cod (3 oz cooked) 449 mg
- tomato (one) 273 mg)

Note: Children 1 year 1000 mg

  2-5   1400 mg
  6-9   1600 mg
  10-18   2000 mg

Sulfur

Sulfur is mineral. It disinfects the blood, protects against toxic substances and helps the body resist bacteria. It protects the cells and is needed for the synthesis of collagen, a principal protein that gives the skin its structural integrity. Acid-forming, it also stimulates bile secretion and is part of the chemical structure of the following:

- Cysteine amino acid: which is the chief protein constituent of the skin. It aids in the production of collagen and helps detoxify.

- Glutathione tripeptide: an antioxidant stores predominantly in the liver, where it detoxifies harmful compounds for their excretion through the bile.

- Methionine amino acid: which assists in digestion and the breakdown of fats. It helps detoxify, is beneficial for chemical allergies, required for the synthesis of collagen, and reduces histamine.

- Taurine amino acid: a key component of bile for the digestion of fats. Necessary for the utilization of potassium and magnesium. Helpful for anxiety. Losses of taurine are associated with overgrowth of candida, stress and zinc deficiency.

Natural Sources of Sulfur

Some natural sources of sulfur are found in brussel sprouts, cabbage, fish, garlic, kale, onions, soybeans and turnips. Sulfur is the key substance that makes garlic the best of all herbs. Horsetail is an herb that has sulfur.

Methylsulfonylmethane "M.S.M"

MSM is an organic form of sulfur. It is non-allergenic and necessary for survival. It can help:

- relieve stress
- relieve constipation

- fight candida
- benefit asthma and arthritis sufferers
- detoxify the body
- strengthen capillary walls and coat and heal intestinal walls
- keep hormones in balance
- relieve food, drug and chemical allergies
- control stomach acidity while maintaining body's normal pH balance
- boost vitamin, mineral and amino acid utilization
- speed the healing of cuts, sores and wounds

Sulfur Testimonies

See a mom's testimony on how MSM helped her son with eczema. This mom's testimony and the research above caused me to try it. I have noticed that my skin is smoother and I'm one more step ahead in the path down recovery. It has helped me, and I would recommend anyone with eczema to try it. This would be among my first priorities as far as supplements are concerned.

Supplements Needed for the Assimilation of Sulfur

Potassium, vitamin B1 (thiamine), vitamin B5 (pantothenic acid) and biotin. See, also, Vitamins and Minerals for Eczema.

Zinc

Zinc helps convert essential fatty acids to prostaglandins and helps in the formation of HCL in the stomach. Necessary for proper functioning of the oil-producing glands. Zinc seems necessary for at least two stages in EFA metabolism, the conversion of linoleic acid to gamma-linolenic acid, and the mobilization of dihomogammalinolenic acid (DGLA) for the synthesis of 1 series PGs. Promotes a healthy immune system and healing of wounds. Not surprisingly, zinc deficits are known to affect hyaluronic acid levels. In a study on rats, among other symptoms, a deficiency in zinc resulted in impaired collagen synthesis.) Protects liver from chemical damage. Needed to maintain proper concentration of vitamin E in the blood. Found in alfalfa, burdock root, cayenne, chamomile, chickweed, dandelion, hops, nettle, parsley, rosehips, sarsaparilla, skullcap and wild yam. Do not take on an empty stomach & not take more than 100mg per day for adults.

Coenzyme Q10

A vitamin like substances. Has the ability to counter histamine and is therefore beneficial for people with allergies. Also beneficial in fighting candidiasis.

Herbs

Aloe Vera

Heals wounds; stimulates cell regeneration; emollient; anti-fungal and antibacterial; good for skin and digestive disorders.

Almond Oil

For dry skin; may soothe itching. Almond oil can be used to cleanse skin.

Alfalfa

Blood & liver purifier. Rich source of nutrients.

Angelica

Anti-inflammatory, aids digestion.

Bilberry (also known as Blueberry)

Strengthens connective tissue; useful for inflammation, stress, anxiety.

Birch

Lessens inflammation and relieves pain. Applied externally is good for sores.

Blackberry Tea

Strengthens the skin and may be used externally to help the eczema.

Black Walnut

Used for fungal infections; aids in digestion; cleanses body of some types of parasites; good also for warts.

Blessed Thistle

Increases stomach secretions; heals liver; alleviates inflammation; purifies blood. Handle with care to avoid toxic skin effects.

Boneset (cousin of the Marigold and Dandelion)

Promotes perspiration, loosens phlegm; cleanses liver and bowels; used for skin diseases and arthritis; anti-inflammatory; calms the body. Long term use not advised.

Borage
Anti-inflammatory, soothing to inflamed/irritated tissues, helps tone and heal nerves; gland balancer; EFAs needed for healthy skin.

Buchu
Used for inflammation and digestive problems.

Burdock
Blood, liver, kidney and lymph purifier; used for skin disorders and cleansing; soothes inflamed or irritated tissues.

Cabbage (Fresh Green Leaves)
Make a poultice, warmed and crushed then layered on the skin under a bandage.

Calendula--Marigold
Topical healer and skin soother; anti-inflammatory; anti-fungal. Calendula or marigold tea or ointment helps relieve itching, blistering and flaking.

Catnip
Relaxant; used for stress; aids digestion and sleep. Good for inflammation, pain and stress.

Cat's Claw
Cleanses intestinal tract, acts as an antioxidant and anti-inflammatory. Not to be used during pregnancy.

Cayenne

Heals tissue; aids digestion and pancreas, spleen; enhances action of other herbs. Useful for arthritis and rheumatism.

Celery Seed

Sedative good for arthritis and nervousness. Not to be used in large amounts during pregnancy.

Chamomile

Sedative, soothing to the nerves, aids digestion; anti-inflammatory Should not be used for long periods of time, or it can produce ragweed allergy. Should not be used by those allergic to ragweed.

Chaparral

Antibacterial; anti-inflammatory; blood purifier; used for arthritis, infections and skin disorders; free radical scavenger; good for skin disorders; poultices can be helpful. Recommended for external use only.

Chickweed

Soothing to inflamed or irritated tissues; used for skin diseases, blood disorders, internal inflammations; chickweed oil or ointment can help relieve itching.

Cinnamon

Enhances digestion and metabolism of fats; fights fungal infection Do not use in large amounts during pregnancy.

Comfrey

Soothing to inflamed or irritated tissues; speeds healing of wounds and skin conditions; beneficial for many skin problems; blood cleanser, heals and soothes bowels; used also for arthritis & asthma External use only.

Dandelion

Cleanses bloodstream; liver detoxifier; increases bile production; mild laxative; used for eczema and rheumatism; combats stress; poultices can be helpful.

Echinacea

Powerful antibiotic, antiviral, antiseptic, anti-inflammatory; blood purifier, immune stimulant. Should not be used by those allergic to plants in the sunflower family.

Elder

Builds blood, cleanses system, eases constipation, fights inflammation, increases perspiration; flowers are used to soothe skin irritations. Do not consume the stems, because they are toxic.

Fenugreek

Lubricates intestines; helps asthma by reducing mucous; good for inflammation.

Feverfew

Anti-inflammatory; used for arthritis and indigestion; aids liver function. Not for use during pregnancy.

Flax

Promotes healthy skin; reduces inflammation.

Garlic

Antibiotic, antiseptic, tones & heals nerves, detoxifier; used for asthma, fungal and bacterial infections.

Gentian

Aids digestion; increases gastric secretions, tones the liver; blood purifier.

Ginger

Promotes perspiration, tones and heals nerves; used for indigestion, cleanses colon; reduces spasms; strong antioxidant and effective antimicrobial for sores and wounds. Don't take in large quantities to avoid stomach upset.

Goldenseal

Antibacterial, antibiotic, antiseptic, anti-inflammatory, tones and heals nerves; cleanses the body; used for liver and gastrointestinal. problems; don't take for more than a week at a time and not to be used during pregnancy. To relieve itching, mix goldenseal root powder with vitamin E, then add a little honey until it's a paste. You can eat it or apply this mixture to the skin. Not for prolonged use during pregnancy.

Gotu Kola

With its effect on connective tissue great value is achieved with the synthesis of collagen, thickening of the skin (a great anti-aging property - as we age our skins become thinner), increasing the tensile strength of the flesh, wound healing, repair of damaged tissue as well as promoting hair and nail growth.

Green Tea

Detoxifies the body, aids digestion. Not to be used in large quantities during pregnancy or while nursing. Don't exceed 2 cups daily.

Hops

Tones and heals nerves; used for insomnia, stress, liver problems, and pain. May help sleep when placed inside the pillowcase.

Horsetail

Promotes healthy skin. Contains sulfur. Used as a poultice accelerates healing of burns and wounds.

Hyssop

Promotes perspiration; used for spleen and bowel problems.

Irish Moss

Soothes inflamed or irritated tissues; used for intestinal problems.

Juniper Berry

Promotes perspiration; aids the pancreas.

Kava Kava

Induces physical and mental relaxation; helpful for anxiety, insomnia, urinary tract infections and stress-related disorders

Can cause drowsiness.

Lavender
Relieves stress; beneficial for skin problems like psoriasis and burns.

Licorice
Soothing to inflamed or irritated tissues, cleanses colon; used for inflammation and stress. Not to be used during pregnancy or to be taken more than a week in a row.

Loganberry Tea
Strengthens the skin and may be used externally to help the eczema.

Marshmallow
Soothes inflamed or irritated tissues and gastrointestinal system.

Milk Thistle
Protects liver; good for adrenal disorders and psoriasis.

Mugwort
Digestant; soothes nerves.

Mustard
Improves digestion; aids in fat metabolism, anti-inflammatory.

Myrrh
Good for skin disorders; antiseptic and disinfectant properties.

Nettle

Anti-allergic, anti-inflammatory; used for arthritis; helps skin complaints associated with poor elimination.

Oregano

Antifungal, anti-allergic, anti-spasmodic, rich in minerals.

Oregon Grape Root

Blood purifier; cleanses and activates the liver; good for many skin conditions.

Papaya Leaf

Contains papain; aids digestion.

Parsley

Used for liver ailments and indigestion; combats stress.

Passion Flower

Sedative, heals and tones the nerves, analgesic, used for insomnia.

Pau D'Arco (Lapacho, Ipe Roxo, Taheebo)

Anti-fungal, blood purifier; used for candida and topically for fungal infections; analgesic, anti-allergic, antimicrobial, anti-inflammatory.

Peppermint

Heals and tones the nerves, sedative, antispasmodic; used for indigestion.

Raspberry Leaf Tea

Strengthens the skin and may be used externally to help the eczema.

Red Clover

Blood purifier; used for skin problems and infection; anti-inflammatory; combats stress.

Rose Hips

Used for stress; source of vitamin C.

Rosemary

Anti-oxidant, antifungal, anti-bacterial.

Sarsaparilla (Smilax)

Hormone balancer, blood & liver purifier; anti-microbial; used for rheumatism; eczema and psoriasis.

Sassafras

Blood purifier, liver cleanser, tonic diaphoretic; for skin disorders.

Skullcap

Tones and heals nerves, sedative, anti-spasmodic; used for nervousness, insomnia.

Slippery Elm

Soothing to inflamed or irritated tissues; used for asthma

Spearmint

Tones and heals nerves, similar to peppermint but milder; used for gas.

St. John's Wort

Blood purifier, immune system stimulant; St. John's Wort oil rubbed into the skin can relieve inflammation and blistering.

Tea Tree Oil

Helps heal fungal infection and virtually all skin conditions
External use only.

Thyme

Promotes perspiration, antiseptic; used for bowel ailments & asthma; eliminates scalp itching and flaking caused by candidiasis.

Turmeric

Protects liver against toxins; antibiotic; anti-inflammatory.
Not to be used in large quantities.

Valerian

Antispasmodic, tones and heals nerves, sedative; used for nervousness, insomnia, stress, anxiety and gas.

Walnut Leaf Tea

Has been used for eczema and externally for skin eruptions.

White Willow

Astringent; used for arthritis and inflammation.

Wintergreen

Relieves pain and inflammation; good for arthritis.

Wood Betony

Heals and tones nerves, sedative, astringent; used for tension, insomnia.

Yarrow

Heals mucous membranes; reduces inflammation, increases perspiration.

Yellow Dock

Astringent; cleans/builds blood; cleanses lymphatic system; used on skin disorders, liver and colon ailments; poultices can help; combined with sarsaparilla, makes a tea for chronic skin disorders.

Yucca

Blood purifier; beneficial for arthritis and inflammatory disorders.

Drugs That Cause Rashes

Go here to see the really long list or just call any pharmacy and ask if a rash could be a side effect of a drug you are using:

http://www.wrongdiagnosis.com/symptoms/rash/side-effects.htm

Hormones

I was studying transepidermal water loss ("TEWL")--that's when water evaporates through the skin--when I started looking at sebum (the oil your skin produces) which keeps TEWL at a minimum. As I studied how sebum is produced by the sebaceous glands, it brought me into the world of hormones.

You see, I had done just about everything I could think of to get my skin glowing again; and, although I was pretty much free of full body eczema, my skin was still generally dry, thin and dull looking. I was having a hard time figuring out why, because I was getting my nutrients, good fats, fat enzymes and drinking plenty of water. Something that clued me in: my clothes were really damp when I took off my thermal suit every night, so I knew my skin was excreting enough water. I had stopped the use of all lotions trying to get my skin to function as the excretion organ it was meant to be instead of treating it like a sponge, but I wasn't getting the oil to come out of my skin, and that's why my skin wasn't glistening and why it continued to dry out easily.

The following is important news about how the different fats we eat affect our hormones and how hormones affect our skin and eczema. MSM sulfur also helps balance hormones.

Ray Peat Ph.D., a physiologist who has worked with progesterone and related hormones since 1968, says that the sudden surge of polyunsaturated oils into the food chain post World War II has caused many changes in hormones. He writes:

Their [polyunsaturated oils] best understood effect is their interference with the function of the thyroid gland. Unsaturated oils block thyroid hormone secretion, its movement in the circulatory system, and the response of tissues to the hormone. When the thyroid hormone is deficient, the body is generally exposed to increased levels of estrogen. The thyroid hormone is essential for making the 'protective hormones' progesterone and pregnenolone, so these hormones are lowered when anything interferes with the function of the thyroid. The thyroid hormone is required for using and eliminating cholesterol, so cholesterol is likely to be raised by anything which blocks the thyroid function.

Testosterone (an androgen hormone) targets the skin and the sebaceous glands where sebum is produced. It combines with the enzyme 5alpha-reductase to produce dihydrotestosterone, which stimulates the sebaceous glands to produce increased volumes of sebum. Sebum is expelled out into the follicular tube. 1/

On mechanism of sebaceous secretion: Downing DT, Strauss JS.

Following the studies of Kligman, most investigators now believe that sebaceous glands function continuously in excreting sebum to the skin surface [7, 8]. Populations of differentiating cells are maintained by mitotic activity both in the peripheral cells of the sebaceous lobules and in aggregations of undifferentiated cells which extend through the body of the lobules. Once formed, and as long as maintained by circulating hormones, each lobule continues to produce a stream of differentiating cells which accumulate sebum as they move towards the sebaceous duct and finally disrupt to release their contents into the pilosebaceous canal. After intradermal injections of 3H-thymidine to label germinative cells during DNA replication, up to 28 days elapse before all labeled cells disappear from the glands. When differentiating cells are labeled with 3H-amino acids, much of the label is lost in 7 days. Likewise, when lipids are labeled with 14C-acetate, the average excretion time for the labeled sebum is 8 days. To this time may be added the renewal time of undifferentiated cells to give an average sebaceous cell transition time of 14 days [15]. From knowledge of the time between synthesis and excretion of sebum, sebum production rates were calculated from the sebum content of punch biopsies. The transit time of sebum in the follicular canals was estimated to be 14 h. Production rates determined in this way agree with those measured by long-term absorption of sebum at the skin surface.

PMID: 7165343 [PubMed - indexed for MEDLINE]

DHEA (For Women and Men)

I knew that topical corticosteroids thinned the skin. However, until I started studying DHEA in-depth as it relates to the skin, I didn't realize that DHEA is extremely necessary for healthy skin and for the functioning of the sebaceous glands. Moreover, I was in for a big awakening to learn that not only does the production of DHEA dramatically reduce with age, but DHEA is also significantly reduced by corticosteroids.

So what is DHEA? Dehydroepiandrosterone (pronounced dee-hi-dro-epp-ee-ann-dro-stehr-own) is a steroid hormone produced in the adrenal gland. It is the most abundant hormone secreted by the adrenal glands. DHEA can also be converted into other steroid hormones, including testosterone and estrogen. After DHEA is made, it goes into the bloodstream, and from there it travels all over the body and goes into our cells where it is converted into male hormones (androgens) and female hormones (known as estrogens). By the way, both sexes need and benefit from both male and female hormones, just in different proportions.

The source material for DHEA powder is derived from wild yams, which are grown commercially. Plant sterols (a class of plant hormones) are extracted from the wild yams. The most common sterol is diosgenin, which has a molecular structure very similar to DHEA. In the laboratory, the diosgenin extract is converted to DHEA by clipping away a few side chains by means of chemical reactions

I had already been very curious about taking male hormones, because data shows that sebaceous glands are stimulated by androgens to produce more sebum. See, also, Hormonal Acne, Androgen, and Sebaceous Glands. That's why teens get hormonal acne and why girls' acne can clear up from taking birth control. The male hormone testosterone keeps skin thick and strong, and only a small amount of androgens is needed to stimulate the oil glands to produce an increase in oil flow from the sebaceous glands. The female hormone estrogen keeps the skin supple by encouraging production of collagen and the NMF hyalauronic acid.

Again, DHEA is a pool from which both male and female hormones are produced, and natural production diminishes with age: 50% reduction by age 50 and 90% by age 90. Women who approach menopause have a decreasing level of estrogen and may experience rapidly thinning and drying skin. According to Professor Carmen Fusco of www.LEF.org, women who take both testosterone and estrogen have really thick skin--48% thicker than women who don't take either hormone. That's important information for people who have eczema, because "new" research says that most people with eczema get it from having thin skin.

Important: zinc increases the size and production of sebaceous gland (good news for us). See, also, this link on zinc's relationship with DHEA stating that zinc deficiency can cause low

DHEA levels. It also supports the synthesis of testosterone and other male hormones.*

Interestingly, I had just begun taking Gotu Kola to help build collagen and stimulate the adrenals. An added benefit: Gotu Kola treats anxiety, because it helps regulate the startle response. Funny thing: Gotu Kola in Chinese means: "The Fountain of Youth," and DHEA is deemed "The Fountain of Youth," because it helps ward of many age-related degenerative diseases; and, in animal studies extended rodent lifespan up to 50%--not only did the animals live longer, they looked younger.

Some studies suggest DHEA may be an effective treatment for major depression when used alone or as an adjunct to antidepressants. DHEA may work by increasing serotonin levels in the brain and blocking the effects of certain stress hormones, such as cortisol.

Re: infants, see: sebum levels during the first year of life.

Natural Progesterone Cream (For Men and Women)

Progesterone acts as an anti-inflammatory agent and regulates the immune response.

First, see this Progesterone and Itch link from an actress who discovered the hard way that hormones were the cause of her extreme itch.

Although progesterone is usually thought of for women, progesterone is needed by men as well (see this article).

A drop in progesterone can cause a concurrent drop in corticosteroid production, leading to a whole other set of symptoms. Progesterone is a major precursor of the important corticosteroid hormones aldosterone and cortisol, made in the adrenal cortex. These corticosteroids are not made via any other hormone pathway. They are responsible for mineral balance, sugar control, and response to stresses of all sorts, including trauma, inflammation, and emotional stress. A lack of corticosteroids can lead to fatigue, immune dysfunction, hypoglycemia, allergies, and arthritis. Not infrequently, progesterone supplementation effectively resolves these problems.

The adrenal cortex is also capable of making progesterone, principally for its precursor role in making corticosteroids, but many women are so stressed out trying to work, raise children, and be wives that by the time they're in their mid to late thirties or early forties their adrenal glands have nothing left to give. My guess is that when Western women stop making progesterone in their ovaries and their adrenal cortex and brain need to pick up 100 percent of that function to produce corticosteroids, there isn't much progesterone left over for other functions, such as balancing estrogen levels. The adrenals of many women in Western cultures are so depleted they can't even make enough progesterone to make the corticosteroids. This may be an important factor in chronic fatigue syndrome, which is so common in women in their mid-thirties and early forties." 1

See, also, how natural progesterone has no side-effects or toxic levels, and here's another great site that talks a lot more about the wonderful use of natural topical progesterone (don't miss it).

Melatonin (For Men and Women)
Melatonin is another beneficial hormone for skin, acting as a protector and antioxidant for skin tissues.

Pregnenolone (For Men and Women)

Pregnenolone is a compound related to DHEA that has recently become the subject of renewed interest. Pregnenolone is made in the body from cholesterol. Pregnenolone is the compound the body uses to make DHEA. Like DHEA, pregnenolone levels drop with age, though not as drastically. Pregnenolone is also the compound from which progesterone is made.

Pregnenolone was used frequently in the 1940's as an anti-inflammatory medicine for arthritis before the advent of more powerful anti-inflammatory drugs such as the corticosteroids. Animal studies of pregnenolone indicate a powerful memory-enhancing effect. It is not yet known how powerful this effect is in humans, but many people are trying pregnenolone since it already has a long safety record. A typical pregnenolone dose for life extension purposes is about 20 milligrams per day. During the 1940's, doses were given for arthritis at about 500 mg. per day, with some of the controlled trials lasting up to two years.

An excellent source for more information about pregnenolone is Pregnenolone: A Practical Guide by Ray Sahelian, M.D. (See the Recommended Reading and Resources section.)

Learn how pregnenolone (abundantly found in coconut oil) is also wonderful for the skin.

Fats and Hormones

Remember there's a huge relationship between fats and hormones, so check out how different fats we eat affect our hormones. Saliva hormone tests are available through your naturopathic doctor.

VI. DETOXIFICATION

Introduction to Detoxification

Some of my trouble was from careless use of household chemicals and lawn and garden chemicals. Before I developed severe full body eczema, I could smell the chemicals and they wouldn't bother me. When my skin was at its worst, just the smell of my dishwasher running would send me running. Detoxifying to reduce sensitivities works. I am no longer careless with chemicals and avoid the ones that bothered me the most like chlorine, car fumes, dishwasher soap.

Avoid letting household chemicals touch the skin and don't breathe the fumes. Probiotics will help detoxify. Drinking water and greens and eating raw fruits and vegetables is helpful to cleanse the body. Herbs that can help detoxify the body are dandelion, garlic and green tea.

Detoxifying With Green Drinks

I learned from an M.D., N.D., Ph.D., after paying $200 for live blood cell analysis that one of the best way to detoxify is with green drinks. I told her that I didn't have a juicer. She said I could just use my blender, so I started blending kale (please see that kale link about how it helps atopic dermatitis and this link on kale, too) and parsley with water. I also mix a handful of parsley (I like Italian parsley), an apple and some carrots in a blender with water and drink that, too. I looked 10 years younger after three months time.

To clean vegetables, use 1 tablespoon of vinegar per gallon of water. Soak for 10 minutes to clean off pesticides. There are other things you can buy to clean them as well.

From Dr. Sandra Cabot - www.liverdoctor.com

The liver is the cleanser and filter of the blood stream and is of vital importance. It is the largest organ in the body and has an enormous amount of blood flowing through it every minute of our lives. It is between 21 - 22.5 cm in its greatest diameter, 15 - 17.5cm in its greatest height and 10 - 12.5 cm in its depth, weighing around 1200 - 1600 gms

The Liver

It is responsible for the production of bile which is stored in the gallbladder and released when required for the digestion of fats.

The liver stores glucose in the form of glycogen which is converted back to glucose again when needed for energy.
It also plays an important role in the metabolism of protein and fats. It stores the vitamins A, D, K, B12 and folate and synthesizes blood clotting factors.

Another important role is as a detoxifier, breaking down or transforming substances like ammonia, metabolic waste, drugs, alcohol and chemicals, so that they can be excreted. These may also be referred to as "xenobiotic" chemicals. If we examine the liver under a microscope, we will see rows of liver cells separated by spaces which act like a filter or sieve, through which the blood stream flows. The liver filter is designed to remove toxic matter such as dead cells, microorganisms, chemicals, drugs and particulate debris from the blood stream. The liver filter is called the sinusoidal system, and contains specialized cells known as Kupffer cells which ingest and breakdown toxic matter.

From Dr. Rebecca Caplan

From a holistic point of view there is little difference in origin between psoriasis and eczema. A similar analysis and regimen is followed with one or two variations.

The Role of the Liver

The liver is the body's main organ of filtration and purification. As the body becomes more toxic the stress on the liver increases, sometimes requiring detoxification of the liver in treatment of skin disease. Often, however, detoxifying the gut will render a separate liver detoxification regimen unnecessary. Sometimes doing a liver detoxification concurrently will hasten the clearing of the skin.

Chemicals, Household Cleansers and Eczema

I cannot stress enough the importance of protecting your breath and your skin from cleaning products. If smells bother you, get a mask to clean until your system can detoxify from the chemical that is bothering it. It's not a good idea to wait until we become chemically sensitive to be careful with chemicals. It is prevention that will help us avoid becoming chemically sensitive. Common sense and following A-B-C's of careful use of chemicals will go very far in preventing chemical sensitization. Remember that the treatment for chemical sensitivity is avoidance. This decreases total body burden and allows for recovery of the overtaxed detoxification system.

Rubbing alcohol, vinegar, lemon and baking soda are friendly cleansers.

See, also, the <u>Gloves</u> section.

Internal Bacteria

Eczema is an Immune System Disorder (atopy), and 75% of your Immune System is found in your Gastrointestinal Tract where 3 to 4 pounds of bacteria reside.

From The American Academy of Dermatology's EczemaNet:

> *"Preliminary studies indicate that probiotics may benefit children with atopic dermatitis."*

NOTICE FOR INFANTS: The normal good intestinal bacteria that reside in healthy infants is not the same as the normal good healthy bacteria that reside in adults. Babies can't handle all good bacteria until they are 4 years of age, because other good bacteria colonies don't normally take up residence until later on in life. Babies are fragile in this way. The only good bacteria that normally inhabits infants is Bifidobacterium infantis.

Now with that understood, see how good bacteria ("probiotics") which are supposed to normally inhabit our gastrointestinal tracts benefit people with eczema and even help prevent eczema in your unborn children. (All are links that can be accessed online at www.eczema.net.)

1. Eczema. A Healthy Breakthrough by Alexander Angelov, M.D.
2. Probiotics for Baby Eczema from Dr. Greene
3. The Beneficial Bacteria and Eczema Connection The Lancet
4. Prebiotic Reduces Eczema in Infants, Healthy Day News
5. Probiotics Cut Atopic Eczema in Infants by Half Skin & Allergy News
6. Eating to Cure Your Eczema, Christine Climer
7. Eczema Patients Lack Natural Antibiotic Web MD
8. Staphylococcus Aureus Colonization in Patients with Atopic Eczema National Institute of Health
9. Probiotics Protect Against Childhood Eczema: 4-year Follow-up.(Clinical Rounds) Pediatric News
10. Probiotics help infants who have eczema, cow's milk allergy: lactobacillus and bifidobacterium Skin & Allergy
11. Probiotics may ameliorate milk allergy eczema: lactobacillus and bifidobacterium.(Clinical Rounds) Pediatric News
12. Probiotics' Benefits in Eczema Affirmed Nutraceuticals International
13. Probiotics Could Reduce Asthma and Eczema in Children. Chemist & Druggist
14. Probiotics Reduced Atopic Eczema Family Practice News
15. Probiotics in the Management of Atopic Eczema. Alternative Medicine Review

Have you heard about the friendly bacteria in yogurt? Lactobacillus acidophilus--which also has anti-fungal properties--is one for example. There are trillions in each person, divided into over four hundred species, most of them living in the digestive tract. Good bacteria help detoxify and protect our bodies, aid in the production of vitamins, enzymes and have antimicrobial effects among other benefits. When the "good guys" are overpowered by the "bad guys", problems like acne, pasty complexion, allergies, bad breath, hair loss, fatigue, auto immune illnesses, depression, heartburn, PMS, digestive disturbances, bloating, intolerances, rheumatoid arthritis and certain nerve disorders can arise. Antibiotics kill both beneficial and harmful bacteria, but probiotics (good bacteria) keep the harmful bacteria in check while at the same time producing natural antibiotics. Good bacteria will also plug up the holes of leaky gut.

International Food Information Council has an extensive article on good bacteria, The Bacteria Museum will teach you how to make food with good bacteria, and see these two great sites as well: Body Ecology Diet and Rejuvenative Foods.

Food Sources of Probiotics
- Yogurt
- Buttermilk
- Kefir
- Tempeh
- Miso
- Kim Chi
- Sauerkraut
- Other "fermented" foods
- Food Sources of Prebiotics
- Flax
- Other whole grains
- Onions
- Greens (especially dandelion greens, but also spinach, collard greens, chard, kale, and mustard greens)
- Berries, bananas, and other fruit
- Legumes (lentils, kidney beans, chickpeas, navy beans, white beans, black beans, etc.)

Bacterial and fungal infections can cause some forms of eczema. With this in mind, inflammation is a process which fights infection. So, steroids (which are anti-inflammatory) may worsen the skin condition if it is caused by bacteria or fungus. (See also the Fungus section.) Neomycin Warning: See the antibiotic ointment allergy section.

Probiotics vs. Antibiotics

Unfortunately, western medicine just treats over-colonization of staphylococcus (common in eczema sufferers) with antibiotics. Don't just try and kill the bad bacteria, but replenish the good bacteria if you have to use an antibiotic. We've learned when we try and kill all the bad bacteria, some are left behind which become more resistant. So, make sure you feed your body beneficial bacteria (topically and orally) to provide an uncomfortable environment for the bad bacteria so that they get pushed out. That's the way to do it. It's like grass, when you kill all the grass, the weeds grow back. Remember: it's the good bacteria that protects us from over colonization of bad bacteria, and beneficial bacteria make natural antibiotics. Also, be aware that many people get rashes from antibiotics.

Effectiveness of Different Kinds of Probiotics

Since people with eczema have trouble breaking down fats, if you are going to supplement, it may be best to start out with a powder as opposed to probiotics that are encapsulated in oil (unless you are taking a lipase enzyme to help digest fat so you can get the benefit of the probiotic that is encapsulated within the oil).

Allergic Component of Eczema

Allergies and Eczema

Eczema can have an allergic component. Remember that probiotics can help with the food allergies associated with eczema. Although nearly any food can cause an allergic reaction, a few foods account for about 90% of reactions. Among adults these foods are peanuts, nuts, fish and shellfish. Among children, they are egg, milk, peanuts, soy and wheat.

Technical Info. We could look at vasoactive intestinal peptide ("VIP") functioning as an anti-inflammatory agent. Or, we could study the anti-inflammatory effects of Interleukin-4, 10 and 14. Or, we could look at C Fibers releasing neurotransmitters, chemicals that regulate nerve impulses, the most important of these C-fiber neurotransmitters being substance P ("SP")--which dilates blood vessels and indirectly activates mast cells. We could investigate the ability to block the SP receptor, either by gene deletion or receptor antagonists and the potent anti-inflammatory analgesic effects that could have, but, we won't do that here.

We will briefly, however, touch upon mast cells and basophils to better understand what's happening. Mast cells are found in tissue, and basophils are found in the bloodstream. Mast cells are responsible for the manifestations of allergy and contribute to skin inflammation. When activated, mast cells release a large number of pro-inflammatory chemicals, including histamine--the amine that causes widening of blood vessels which irritate nerve fibers in the skin and cause redness and swelling of the skin.

From a brochure by NEASE:

"We know that AD is a disease of inflamed skin. That

*inflammation is a result of various cells coming into the
skin and causing itching, redness and swelling. Those
cells come from the person's bone marrow, then they
travel through the blood stream to the target tissues: the
skin in AD, the nose in hay fever, the lungs in asthma.
Something makes these cells over-react. They generate
too much inflammation and they don't stop. Maybe that's
the cause of the disease--cells that create too much
damage when they turn on and they don't turn off the way
they should. We don't know the reason for the defective
"on/off switch." We can only try to control AD by
preventing the "on" trigger. Things that turn "on" the
switch are called trigger factors."*

Excess inflammation? Is the body right? Considering all
the inflammatory diseases, I think that in most cases there is a
reason for the "excess" inflammation and don't believe it is mostly
due to defective "on/off switches" (that would be too many
defective switches). In my case, I also had some candida
overgrowth and part of my problem was a pepped up immune
system that was trying to fight off the yeast infection. Most
doctors will tell you that an overgrowth of candida in the GI tract
is rare. But, since birth control pills, steroids, antibiotics, and a
high sugar and carbohydrate encourage overgrowth of candida, my
bet is that many people have too much candida. Asthma, allergies,
arthritis, chronic fatigue syndrome can also be symptoms of an
overgrowth of candida.

See if an anti-candida diet improves your condition by
reducing sugars and yeasts.

Magnesium, Hydrochloric Acid and Digestion

Magnesium is needed to reduce histamine levels. In the
book Encyclopedia of Natural Medicine, the authors note that food

allergies are usually associated with low hydrochloric acid levels and poor digestion. The authors' rationale for this is that low stomach acid leaves food undigested and fermenting in the intestinal tract. This fermentation causes gas, bloating and stomach upset, the symptoms of irritable bowel syndrome. Undigested and fermented food causes the body to raise histamine levels, which produce allergic reactions. This is why people take antihistamines for allergies, to lower histamine levels.

Low stomach acid levels reduce levels of beneficial intestinal bacteria which is needed for absorption of magnesium. When lab rats are deprived of magnesium, a wide variety of studies have noted that they develop allergy like symptoms. Their ears turn red and they develop skin problems. Rats with magnesium deficiencies have increases in histamine levels. They also have raised levels of white blood cell counts. Mg deficiency has been implicated in allergies and allergic skin reaction in many studies on humans, too. Variations of allergies, skin allergies, and raised white blood cells have all been noted as features of many chronic disorders.

My Internal Experience

With my eyes swollen almost closed for 2 months, along with the bridge of my nose, my cheeks became so red until golden liquid bubbled through. My face was in a cycle of inflammation.

I used internal and external steroids and antihistamines. They reduced some symptoms, but they left the root of the problem untouched. The topical steroid caused cortisone-induced rosacea (red dots), and the internal steroid (prednisone) caused weight gain and bruising. They didn't break the cycle of inflammation.

Since my face was swelling, I thought of it as an allergic response. I learned that some allergies involved with eczema are food allergies. I was tested by a allergist for all the common allergens, but nothing came back as positive. My last words to the allergist were, "So, we can safely say it's an allergic reaction to something, but we just don't know to what, right?" He said, "Right."

Here's some information about testing the blood for delayed hypersensitivity with regard to food allergies. Many in the naturopathic profession believe that in 65% of cases, this can be the managing key. Most dermatologists and immunologists, however, won't agree with the naturopaths regarding this kind of testing ... dermatologists says it's mostly genetic and immunologists just do the instant skin tests and don't use this blood test for delayed hypersensitivity. I side with the naturopaths ... it helped me. See: Immuno Laboratories

Fasting

The only thing I could think of was ridding my body of the allergen that I couldn't pinpoint. I thought about fasting. It takes 4 days for foods to leave our system. I began to fast to clear my body of any allergens. The idea of fasting is that since the body isn't busy digesting food, it can work on eating the other things inside the body that don't belong (like allergens in the blood).

I began to get better the very first day while fasting. The second day my eyes were not swelling as they had done every day for the 2 months prior. Kind of like how the clouds clear and the sun shines, the red patches were clearing and the white skin was showing again. Two months of swelling eyes had come under control. I was happy that it didn't take any medicine to do that. The cycle of inflammation was broken.

I didn't do a total fast; I just fasted in the daytime and ate uncooked fruits and vegetables in the evening. The Fasting Center International has more information about fasting for allergies. My immunologist says he doesn't believe it's good, but I do because it's in the Bible and because those who have studied it say it is good to help the body get rid of toxins and allergens.

The Master Cleanser (Not Recommend for Candida)

This is a wonderful fast by Stanley Burroughs. It cleanses the body, for "As the lymphatic glands become clogged, they are no longer able to assimilate and digest even the best of foods. As we cleanse our bodies and free our cells and glands of toxins that clog and paralyze our assimilation, we free our various organs and processes to do their proper jobs." The Master Cleanser book is found in health food stores for about $6.00. I went on this fast for 10 days. "Because it is a complete balance of minerals and vitamins, one does not suffer the pangs of hunger." The caution is to be careful on how to come off of a fast (slowly and with the right kind of foods is extremely important), or the body can go into shock ... could be fatal coming off a long fast incorrectly, so always consult with a professional if you're going to fast.

My External Experience

I hear people say, "Well, I've been using that for years and it has never bothered me, so it can't possibly be that!" Sometimes it takes a while for people to become sensitized to a chemical. It's a good idea to switch products now and then so we don't become sensitized to the chemicals (like alternating foods ... same concept ... so we don't become sensitive to them). The treatment for chemical sensitivity is avoidance, this decreases total body burden and allows for recovery of the overtaxed detoxification system.

Candida

Here are some problems that can be symptoms of a systemic candida yeast infection:

- Eczema; severe itching; night sweats; skin that's hot to the touch;
- Burning tongue, white tongue, thrush (yeast infection in baby's mouth) & diaper rash; Dandruff (P. ovale yeast); loss of body hair; warts;
- Digestive disorders like indigestion, constipation, diarrhea, abdominal pain, gastritis, bowel movement followed by white discharge; loss of appetite, weight fluctuations;
- Menstrual problems; frequent bladder and vaginal infections;
- Inflammatory joint pain, heel spurs; arthritis; muscle problems, back pain;
- Emotional problems, panic attacks, irritability, sudden mood swings; insomnia;
- Cravings for sugar and breads; food sensitivities
- Increased chemical sensitization to rubber, petroleum products, tobacco, exhaust fumes and chemical odors;
- Memory loss; headaches;
- Bad breath, sore, bleeding gums or dry mouth, canker sores; persistent sore throat or nagging cough;
- Tearing or chronically inflamed eyes; pain or fluid in the ears; recurrent ear infections
- Adrenal problems.
- Things that can attribute to candida overgrowth are antibiotics, birth control pills, corticosteroids and a diet that is high in sugar and carbohydrates.

Genova Diagnostics Laboratory provides testing, and remember that good bacteria will help this condition.

Celiac Disease and Gluten Sensitivity

Celiac comes from the Greek word meaning "suffering of the bowels." When people with celiac disease consume gluten-- which is a protein found in wheat, rye, oats and barley--the villi in the small intestine are damaged and prevent the absorption of many important nutrients.

Eczema As a Symptom of Celiac Disease

Chronic tissue inflammation and eczema can be a symptom of Celiac disease, and skin disorders in people with this disease can be cleared by cutting down or eliminating gluten from the diet.1 Most of the complications of celiac disease are due to malabsorption. The absorption of vitamin B-12 was shown to be significantly decreased in infants with celiac disease.

My naturopathic physician says every time he eats wheat, he gets eczema on his fingers. I remember when I cut out breads for 8 months, my skin improved a whole lot. If you haven't tried avoiding gluten before, you might consider cutting out the wheat, rye, oats and barley for a couple of weeks and see how your condition improves.

Here's a great page from Wikipedia on The Gluten-Free Diet. See, also, the Watery, Itchy Blisters section.

What People Eat Instead

- Rice
- Tapioca
- Potatoes
- Vegetables
- Corn
- Most beans

Wheat Allergy Letter

Hi Christina,

I had eczema from about 5 years of age until 34. I suffered terribly with cracked and bleeding hands. Many medications and therapies over the years never worked. In fact, one medication further depleted the integrity of my skin. In my 20's (in the mid to late 80's) I began to believe (intuitively) that the cause of and cure to my eczema would prove to be internal – not externally applied. I began reading about skin and vitamins. The Dr.'s I saw did not offer much assistance, humbly admitting to being stumped and knowing little about implementing vitamin therapies. By the time I was in my 30's my skin was so terrible that I had to hold my right hand in a closed position. Attempting to open this hand and spread my finger would result in instant cracking and bleeding. My left hand was not nearly as severe. (And I am right handed). Today I'm pretty good using both hands for most tasks (except writing) due to years using my left hand b/c the right hand was incapable.

So on to the happy ending to all the pain – by chance I discovered my insensitivity (or allergy) to wheat. A friend asked me to try the Atkins diet with her & being about 10 lbs. overweight at the time, I agreed. Within 6 weeks I was completely free of the eczema – that, to me, was a miracle. My only confirmation is that I did try to eat Pizza and other wheat products after my friend declared we were no longer dieting; and sure enough, the eczema started to come back. I searched the web (by this time it is 1998) and found postings from people who made the same claim to eczema/wheat. I promptly stopped consuming wheat product again and haven't eaten any since. I have remained eczema free; and it took a few years, but the scarring has diminished and my fingerprints have returned.

Joan

Free Radicals

Medical and scientific researchers are convinced that uncontrolled free radical activity in the body is directly associated with a number of health problems. Dry skin, allergies, asthma, inflamed tissues, psoriasis, stress damage, wrinkling of the skin, skin cancer and liver damage are just a few of over 60 diseases/disorders in which free radicals have been implicated.

To help understand, electrons normally come in pairs; a free radical is an atom or molecule with an unpaired electron. This unpaired electron in a free radical causes it to collide with other molecules so it can steal an electron from them, which changes the structure of these other molecules and causes them to also become free radicals. This can create a chain reaction in which the structure of millions of molecules are altered.

How do free radicals get into our bodies? From "within", as the natural by-products of ongoing biochemical reactions occurring in normal metabolic functions, in the detoxification processes and in immune system defense. From "without", free radicals come from food, water, drugs, medicines, radiation, pesticides, air pollutants, solvents, fried foods and alcohol.

But, free radical scavengers (antioxidants) neutralize the activity of these free radicals. Antioxidants work by donating or "sacrificing" an electron to the free radical, which then becomes paired with the formerly unpaired electron, thereby stabilizing and, in effect, eliminating the free radical. Although the body will produce anti-oxidant defenses, it also makes great use of nutrients and minerals such as vitamins E, C and beta-Carotene and the minerals selenium and zinc.

Now, a whole new subclass of bioflavonoid compounds called flavenes has been discovered. These flavan molecules are called Oligo Proantho Cyanidins ("OPCs"). As free-radical scavengers, these substances are 50 times more powerful than Vitamin E and at least 20 times stronger than Vitamin C. OPCs are many times more effective as free radical neutralizers than anything previously discovered. Dr. Masquelier named his new find pycnogenols (which means to condense into one).

Active pycnogenols have been isolated from many plants that are natural food sources like apples, hawthorn berries, cocoa beans, quince, cherries, grapes, raspberries, blackberries, cranberries, sorghum, strawberries, beans, hops and rose hips. Pycnogenols have been found to be present in many red wine. For me, unfortunately, it's the sulfites in the red wines that my body doesn't like.

Electrons and Eczema

Why People Like Sitting in the Sun, by the Beach, in the Mountains, and By Waterfalls ...

Certain places in nature seem almost magical. You feel wonderful when you're on a beach with crashing surf, next to a rushing waterfall, or high in the mountains. There is one simple reason. The air in these places is supercharged with negative ions. These naturally occurring atomic particles have been demonstrated to help produce a number of beneficial effects in human beings, including increased energy, enhanced ability to handle stress, keener awareness, greater dream recall and an overall sense of tranquility.

Places we find refreshing such as mountains, waterfalls and seashores - where traditional health resorts are situated - are found to have high concentrations of negative ions. But, high levels of positive ions often make us feel uncomfortable.

What are Air Ions?

An ion is a molecule that has gained or lost an electron. Positive air ions are molecules that have lost an electron; a negative air ion is generally a molecule of oxygen with an extra electron.

Molecules with extra electrons form negative ions, and have a positive effect on the environment. They neutralize odors and contribute to the clean air and fresh smell we find in non-industrial sparsely populated areas. Positive ions are produced by car and factory exhausts, cigarette smoke, dust, soot and other pollutants.

If the electrical charge was negative, it imparted a positive feeling of health and vitality. If it carried a positive charge, people (and animals for that matter) felt negative and suffered the symptoms of the notorious oppressive winds.

The Calm After the Storm

Many people find the atmosphere before a storm is 'heavy' and oppressive. This has been attributed to the high levels of positive ions that build up in the air, which are also believed to be the trigger of "storm-sensitivity" in asthmatics. Certainly, in laboratory conditions, similar symptoms could be stimulated in subjects exposed to abnormally high positive ion levels. Immediately after the storm, the air feels clean and refreshed, filled with negative ions.

Environments

In our modern life, we have created an environment that virtually eliminates negative ions from the atmosphere. Negative ions are readily attracted to airborne particles. (This is how they clean the air - by attaching to particles of dust, pollen, smoke, thus giving them a 'static' charge which pulls them to the ground.) So while there is a higher concentration of ions in the countryside, as you move into towns and cities, the dirt and pollution causes the level to drop dramatically. Pollution from car exhausts, cigarette smoking, overcrowding and even breathing, all contribute to this. Ironically, today's air conditioned buildings, vehicles and planes frequently become supercharged with harmful positive ions because the metal blowers, filters and ducts of air-conditioning systems strip the air of negative ions before it reaches its destination. In addition, fluorescent lighting, electrical and electronic equipment, television screens, and static producing, man-made fibers in carpets, clothes and curtains all reduce the level of negative ions and increase the positive.

Health and Electrons

The effect of this negative ion depletion varies from person to person; the least fortunate can suffer migraine, asthma and severe depression. Most authorities agree that ions act on our capacity to absorb and utilize oxygen. Negative ions in the bloodstream accelerate the delivery of oxygen to our cells and tissues. Positive ions slow down the delivery of oxygen, producing symptoms markedly like those in anoxia, or oxygen starvation. The body chemical serotonin, linked with mood and stress, is also influenced by air ion levels. Too many positive ions make the levels rise, causing stress and discomfort. Increasing the negative ion concentration helps bring relief. Researchers believe that negative ions may stimulate the reticulo-endothelial system, a group of defense cells in our bodies which marshal our resistance to disease.

Interestingly, it was discovered that in many people, the body's initial respond to positive ions is to produce adrenaline and noradrenaline - the "fight or flight" hormones - which produces short-term euphoria but eventually leads to a condition of exhaustion. (It is this condition that is thought to affect insects and animals into restless activity as the positive ions build up before a storm.) The research also showed that exposure to positive ions can trigger an over-production of histamine, which most people will immediately recognize as the body chemical that aggravates allergies. Statistically it was found that 25% of the population are quite strongly affected by levels of ions in the air. Of the remainder, 50% are affected considerably, although 25% do not appear sensitive at all.

Negative Charges

Quick background: In the center of an atom is a nucleus. The nucleus is the bulk of the atom. It contains the proton, which is positively charged and the neutron, which has no charge. This is what gives the atom its weight. Around the nucleus are negatively charged electrons orbiting in circles. We know that two magnets will attract each other ... the nucleus is a positive magnet while the electrons are negative magnets (this keeps them close together).

From Magnotherapy & Electromagnetic Energy: "We may not think of ourselves as electric. Yet most of us are aware of the electric impulses that spark our nervous system particularly those that have been measured in our brains and those that regulate our heartbeat. We're less aware of the fascia system of connective tissues in our bodies (crystalline arrays of collagen fibers). These tissues are piezoelectric. This means they generate electric fields when compressed that's every time the body moves, even when a gland secretes. Sheets of these fascia connectors cover all muscles, organs, and structures of the body. They form a semi-conductive 'electric' network throughout the body. "

Diseased, infected, and injured tissue can be shown to all be positively charged. The resulting electromagnetic positive signal is sent to the brain through the nervous system and the brain in turn returns an electromagnetic negative signal. It is this negative energy that is necessary for governing the healing process. The negative energy reinforcements are sent from other areas of the body.

Thus positive energy irritates the body stimulating negative charged response. This is our natural defense system and will benefit us unless the positive energy persists (resulting in persistent pain) or sufficient negative energy is not available (due to fatigue or unhealthy bodies).

There's also less known about the meridian system. Along this system are many energy centers or trigger points that control or direct bodily functions. Over 1,000 such centers have been identified. They are electric in nature. Alternative treatment methods such as yoga, homeopathy, massage, chiropractic, magnotherapy and acupuncture all use these points. Dr. Pawluk says that he frequently uses magnets instead of needles on meridian acupuncture points.

Negative Charge in Minerals

Lacking vitamins, the body can use minerals; but, without minerals, vitamins cannot be utilized. The colloidal minerals (that come in liquid form) have a natural negative electrical charge. This has two very important benefits: it greatly increases the transport and bioavailability of other nutrients gotten from foods and/or vitamins and other supplements, and it ill attract toxins and heavy metals from the body and flush them out.

Electrons and Free Radicals

Free radicals destroy electrons and antioxidants replace them. Humans have a higher concentration of electrons than other organisms. The electrons in cells serve as the resonance system for the sun's energy. Light waves are in accord with humans and it's no coincidence that people love the sun. This concentration of the sun's energy is improved when foods rich in electrons are consumed.

Electrons in Food

"Foods containing essential fatty acids, especially unrefined organic flax oil, are a rich source of electrons. Electrons have a negative charge and orbit around nuclei, which have a positive charge. Electrons in motion produce an electrical charge, which in turn produces a magnetic field. When they both connect an electrical current is produced. It is this current that keeps the heart ticking and the blood circulating."

From Dynawave Medical Technologies

"Injured tissue exhibits an increase in bio-electrical resistance due to blood and oxygen depletion. The transport of nutrients to and wastes from the cells becomes compromised resulting in pain and inflammation. Typical bio-electric voltage levels of healthy cells switch between -90 and + 20 mill volts when depolarization occurs. Injured cells are not able to fully depolarize when bio-electric resistance increases. This results in a delay of the body's own ability to begin the healing process until the tissue has recovered substantially from trauma."

VII. STRESS MANAGEMENT

Stress and Anxiety

Hong Kong's Dept. of Health has an eczema web site that states, "Avoid unnecessary ... emotional stress." The American Academy of Dermatology's section on atopic dermatitis states, "Seek advice from your dermatologist about dealing with ... emotional upsets which make the condition worse." The Merck Manual's section on atopic dermatitis states, "Intolerance to primary irritants is common, and emotional stress ... commonly cause exacerbations."

Are You Under Great Stress?

Though eczema stressed me out, dealing with a stressful relationship terrifically helped clear up the eczema. There is an excellent book on healthy boundaries relationships. It's called Boundaries by Henry Cloud and John Townsend. The analogy: as long as a fish is in chlorinated water, no matter what you feed him, he'll still be sick. Learn about healthy boundaries in relationships. Very fun, huge and life saving. Teach your kids ...

How I Attacked Anxiety After It Attacked Me

My eczema was so unbearably itchy that within a year's time I worked my way up to twenty antihistamines daily; that is, 3 every 3 hours and probably enough to put a horse to sleep. Since the Benadryl wasn't helping anyway, I suddenly stopped taking it.

Soon after, I was experiencing severe adrenalin rushes that wouldn't turn off, otherwise known as the "fight or flight response" or panic attacks. Although the eczema was bad, the attacks were worse ... couldn't breath, got sick, felt like I needed to die.

Doctors told me that I would have to stay on anti-panic attack medicine my whole life. Even with the medicine I was still plagued with attacks. Once again, I had to beat the odds and figure out how to get better despite the hopelessness. I thank Lucinda Bassett, Founder of The Midwest Center for Stress and Anxiety, Inc., for her book From Panic to Power. I'm forever grateful. Now, I don't take anti-anxiety medicine and no more attacks either. I learned anti-stress coping techniques that I'd like to share with you to help curb the stress before it aggravates the eczema.

Another book that helps with self-esteem, emotional anchorage and security is a book by Steven Covey called "7 Habits of Highly Effective People." I loved it. It helped me a lot.

There are amazingly wonderful free short videos by Doctors Henry Cloud and John Townsend which can be found here: http://cloudtownsend.com.

Top Twelve Coping Skills

1. Over intellectualizing and overanalyzing is not so good. "What if's" and "I should have's" are not good when they are negative. The first is anticipatory anxiety and the latter is being over reflective. Worrying about the future and the past can be unhealthy. Stay in the present. If you must think forward or reflect, set a time limit.

2. If you need to lecture, make it short and not drawn out. Then, the rule of thumb is to give 10 times that amount of praise.

3. Be compassionate, patient and gentle with yourself. Stop thinking, saying and doing things that make you feel bad, anxious or upset with yourself. I used to think that talking to one's self was for kooks. Now I know that talking to yourself in an encouraging way is key in a healthy thought life. Be your own best friend by the way you talk to yourself; be nice to yourself in your thought life. Your value isn't gotten from what others think about you (not even from what you think about yourself), because God's truth is that you are great and you are loved.

4. Go ahead and have high standards, but steer clear of perfectionism.

5. When making decisions, remember that it's not a science and that you can always modify.

6. Taking responsibility for our feelings instead of blaming them on something else allows us to be in control of our feelings.

7. Lean to under react. I thought that this would be frustrating; but, it actually is kind of fun, because you end up feeling better. It does get easier with time.

8. Learn about healthy boundaries in relationships. When to say "yes" and when to say "no" without feeling guilty to take control of your life. <u>Boundaries</u>.

9. Being unable to forgive people is stressful. Forgiving and trusting are two different things, so just because you forgive doesn't mean you should trust .. trust is earned, but no sense in torturing yourself when the enemy is oblivious to your pain anyway. Remember Cinderella's, "In my own little corner and my own little world, I can be whatever I want to be" ... angry or happy or sad or whatever, may as well be happy. (lol)

10. Tone down on "attentional bias," (a tendency to stress our supposed social stumbles) and "interpretational bias," (a habit of picking up neutral cues from other people and interpreting them as evidence of failing socially).

11. Exercise is great.

12. Vitamins and herbs are helpful.

Did you know that panic disorder and multiple chemical sensitivity may be linked to enzyme deficiencies?

Cortisol - Nothing Helps Regulate Cortisol Better than Sleep, So Get Your Rest ...

Cortisol (hydrocortisone) is a powerful hormone manufactured by the adrenal gland. When it is within normal levels it helps individuals cope with normal everyday stress. When manufactured in large amounts or found at elevated levels as a result of chronic stress, cortisol becomes a killer, affecting practically all cells, tissues and organs in the human body. Elevated levels of cortisol have been reported in the literature with regards to eczema.

In stress there is a vigorous release of corticotrophin releasing hormone (CRH), which leads to the release of cortisol. CRH stimulates the mast cells to secret chemicals, including histamine and interleukins. Histamine widens blood vessels, causing them to become more permeable, thus allowing white blood cells to leak through. The interleukin then attracts the blood cells toward the skin tissue. The white cells then settle in areas under the skin, and together with other mast cell secretions cause symptoms, including skin inflammation, scales, and itch.

Cycle of Stress

When stress causes an organism to secrete glucocorticoids repeatedly, the regulation of the system stops working as well, and the organism starts to hyper secrete glucocorticoids even under non-stressful circumstances. If stress can influence immune function (and it does), then the brain must be able to influence the immune system, since stressors are first perceived in the brain. Most scientists now know accept the power of psychological variables to modulate stress physiology.

Train Yourself to Focus on the Good for Better Health

You may see "How stress and thoughts and feelings affect the immune and hormonal systems of the body" by visiting The Institute of HeartMath.

See, also, the Anti-Stress Coping Skills section.

Premenstrual Syndrome

First, see: NIH's report: on Estrogen dermatitis.

Department of Obstetrics and Gynecology, Cumhuriyet University, School of Medicine, Kadin Hastaliklari Anabilim Dali, Sivas, Turkey.

The aim of the present study was to evaluate the estrogen dermatitis of women who have chronic skin disorders with exacerbations or premenstrual dermatitis in a cyclic pattern. Twenty-three women exhibiting skin disorders of pruritus, urticaria, eczema, papulovesicular eruption, hirsutism-acne with hyperpigmentation (hirsutism and/or its related disorders such as acne) and 18 healthy control subjects were included in the study. Sensitivity to estrogen was described in 14 of 23 women. Of the 14 estrogen sensitive women, nine had a premenstrual flare of their skin lesions and five had a chronic dermatitis with *exacerbations. In the evaluation of endocrine profile, mean serum testosterone and LH levels of the patient group were significantly higher than controls (2.814 +/- 0.839 vs. 1.561 +/- 0.645 nm/l, P < 0.001; 10.843 +/- 2.538 vs. 4.539 +/- 1.215 IU/l, P < 0.0001). The LH/FSH ratio of the patient group was also significantly higher than controls (1.765 +/- 0.329 vs. 0.810 +/- 0.0116, P < 0.0001). Mean serum progesterone level of the patient group was significantly lower than the control group (0.499 +/- 0.201 vs. 0.977 +/- 0.396 ng/ml, P < 0.001). Hyperandrogenism and anovulation were the two more common outcomes in the patient group. Skin lesions of estrogen sensitive women were all cured with the administration of tamoxifen 20 mg daily for 7 days premenstrually. PMID: 9076430*

[PubMed - indexed for MEDLINE]

About 75% of women experience some kind of premenstrual syndrome. Anxiety and skin eruptions are the two symptoms we'll name here. Just like some women might break out with a little acne when they have their monthly, many women with eczema report that their eczema flares up with their cycle. It makes sense, considering what the stress hormone can do to our immune system. Help balance your hormones with wild yams (progesterone).

There are a number of supplements recommended for eczema that are also recommended for PMS. Among them are essential fatty acids and vitamins and minerals such as magnesium, B vitamins, vitamin E, lecithin, vitamin A, vitamin C and zinc.

Regarding diet, eating plenty of fresh fruits and vegetables, drinking plenty of water, and cutting down on red meats, junk food and dairy products may be helpful.

For a lot more on hormones, see the DHEA section.

Lack of Sleep from Itching

Itching in the night seems to be the main problem here. I noticed that I itched the most after showering or bathing, so I tried not to do that right before bed. Sometimes it was from something I put on the skin, so I rinsed it off with cold water and used something else.

If you suspect certain foods, avoid them before bed for a while and see if that helps. See, also, the Anti-Itch section. I bought a cold pack made of blue gel. I kept it in the freezer and used it to help relieve itching at night. It comes with a cover that is soft and keeps the skin from getting wet. It was helpful, too.

The Clothing section may be helpful with regards to pajamas and bedding that may contribute to itching.

Sleep Aids

Recommended for eczema and insomnia are magnesium and B vitamins. Probiotics also have a calming effect on the body. Bananas, almonds, figs and dates contain tryptophan, which promotes sleep; and, herbs helpful for eczema and insomnia are hops, kava kava, passionflower, skullcap and valerian root. It's always best not to rely on one root, but to switch around.

Support Groups

I used to be a member of a huge eczema group on the Net. I don't belong to one anymore, because I had a bad experience with the people who ran it. It seemed reckless.

Support Groups Offline and In Person Through Meetup.com

Regarding face to face support groups for eczema, I've found that they are rare. We can change that. Publicity is the key. Place ads in your local newspapers to form support groups for people with eczema. Write your local public radio and public television stations announcing the formation of the support group and give a phone number for people to call. Call the local hospitals and dermatologists offices asking for permission to place a flyer in their buildings, again, announcing the formation of a local support group for people with eczema.

Before meeting, the person forming the support group should contact other support groups in the area and get their ideas on how a support group functions. Maybe the group could start out with a prayer. Some advice is probably needed to help the organizational flow of the meeting; others support groups may be able to simply explain how they hold their meetings.

Some Thoughts About Support Groups

The person forming the support group is not responsible for teaching the group how to get better.

The progress of the group should be in terms of building relationships where they feel comfortable enough to discuss their concerns.

Having positive thinking people there is so important. Storms in life come to all, but how you take the storm depends a lot on the attitude. A focus of the group should be on handling the stress.

They must remember that they are there to support and encourage each other. I don't think it should be looked upon as a class of some sort; rather, it is a place to meet friends who are going through the same thing.

VIII. INFANT AND CHILD ECZEMA

Seven Areas to Consider

1. What is the pH of the formula your baby is drinking? We need to be alkaline internally. Regarding infant formulas, metabolic acidosis is common in babies fed cows' milk-based formula. Eczema can be an emergency expulsion of acid toxins through the skin, and this is one huge reason why so many babies have eczema and then outgrow it when they get off the formula. Also, if the mother's milk is too acidic, so will the baby be. Soy can be debatable too (it has enzyme inhibitors). Go with goat's milk for infant formula and for kids (it's alkaline). If we are acidic inside, we get sick. Midwives make their own formula.

2. Go to the probiotics link, learn about good bacteria, how the lack of it may attribute to eczema in unborn children, and how infants, children and adults can clear up eczema with the addition of it. From Dr. Greene's web site: "Many children with eczema have flare-ups triggered by what they eat or drink. In one

fascinating study, a group of children who received Lactobacillus had significant improvement of their eczema within one month."

Babies can only handle the Bifidobacterium infantis bacteria (that's the good bacteria that normally resides in the healthy infants. That is why there are probiotics just for infants. The Life Start product found in the Eczema Mall under "Probiotics" is just for infants. Midwives develop their own infant formulas and add LifeStart to it. Baby aren't ready for other bacteria until they are four years old, because the good bacteria that normally resides in the GI tract of an adult is not the same as for babies. If there is an infection, babies could handle acidophilus for a week, but that's about it, and only under the supervision of a professional. Again, babies aren't developed enough for other bacteria until they are 4 years of age. It's a very different story with adults, though.

3. What is the pH of the products (skin and hair) that you are using on the children. Many products are alkaline, destroying the acid mantle ... and that's one reason many babies suffer from fungal diaper rashes. We need to protect the acid mantle.

4. Is the infant eating lots of cereal containing gluten, or is the child eating a lot of pizza, breads, bagels ... foods containing gluten? Not saying take the pizza away from kids but am saying try thin crust and maybe substitute tortillas for bread and many food, dairy and gluten allergies are from an imbalance of bacteria in the GI tract. See, also, the most common allergenic foods in the Diet section.

5. Is the infant or child getting essential fatty acids like those in flaxseed oil? I dip my tortillas in flax oil (celtic salted), and my son and I both love it ... hard to get oil down any other

way. Also, crushed flaxseeds mixed with Grade B maple syrup are a nice tasty treat.

6. Stress is an issue. Please see the <u>Stress</u> section for more.

7. The feeling of clothing on the skin is significant, so please see the <u>Clothing</u> section and cut off all the tags (because they itch and feel terrible).

If you can change any one of these, it could make all of the difference. The nice thing about it is that since there are so many things we can do, you don't need to be perfect in anything.

NIH Note: Sebum levels during the first year of life. (See, also, <u>DHEA</u> section.)

See, also, <u>The Inflammation Free Diet Plan.</u>

IX. CLOSING COMMENTS

I probably could have said just drink your water, eat your fruits and veggies, cut down on junk food, get your good fats and enzymes and your good bacteria, too; and, watch out for gluten; and, make sure you're not careless with chemicals, and try to preserve your skin's acid mantle by restoring the proper pH; and, don't let people treat you bad, and train yourself to think about the good things so that you have more peace in your life; but, maybe you wouldn't have realized how important all that is ... until you went over it piece by piece and detail by detail. (smile)

You can get better. Take baby steps and don't be a perfectionist, but never give up hope ... because you don't have to. Remember, every little thing you do will help your body's ecology. It is not about a defective body, it's about heading in the right direction no matter where you are coming from. All these things you've read about here point in one direction: to better emotional and physical health.

Here's to you, you can do it. I know you can. It happened to me.